CONQUER PAIN:
The Natural Way

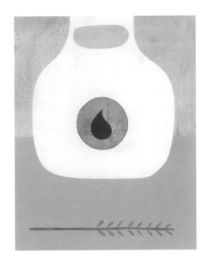

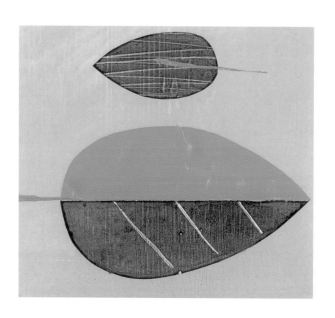

CONQUER PAIN:
The Natural Way

How to break
the pain cycle
and regain control
of your life

LEON CHAITOW

DUNCAN BAIRD PUBLISHERS

LONDON

Conquer Pain
Leon Chaitow

First published in the United Kingdom and Ireland in 2002 by
Duncan Baird Publishers Ltd
Sixth Floor, Castle House
75–76 Wells Street
London W1T 3QH

Conceived, created and designed by Duncan Baird Publishers

Managing Editor: Judy Barratt
Editor: James Hodgson
Managing Designer: Manisha Patel
Designer: Rachel Cross
Commissioned artwork: Sarah Ball
Commissioned medical artwork (p.144): Debbie Maizels
Commissioned photography: Matthew Ward

British Library Cataloguing-in-Publication Data:
a CIP record for this book is available from the British Library

ISBN: 1-903296-57-9

1 3 5 7 9 10 8 6 4 2

Typeset in Bembo and Trade Gothic
Colour reproduction by Scanhouse, Malaysia
Printed by Imago, Singapore

publisher's note

Conquer Pain is not intended as a replacement for professional medical treatment and advice. The Publisher and
Author cannot accept responsibility for any damage incurred as a result of any of the therapeutic methods contained in
this work. If you are suffering from a medical condition and are unsure of the suitability of any of the therapeutic methods
in this book, or if you are pregnant, it is advisable to consult a medical practitioner. Essential oils must be diluted in
a base oil before use. They should not be taken internally and are for adult use only.

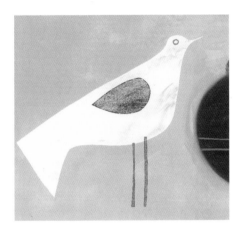

This book is dedicated to my wife
Alkmini with love and thanks

CONTENTS

INTRODUCTION

Pain is a universal experience – one that has more descriptive words attached to it than perhaps any other sensation. However, the way that different people cope with pain can vary greatly. One of the main aims of this book is to show you how to approach *your* pain positively, in a way that will enable you to gain control over it and to lead as normal a life as possible.

All too often we use our pain as an excuse to retreat from performing everyday tasks, which leads to a spiral of inactivity, increased disability and loss of self-confidence. However, it is possible to reverse this tendency – a crucial first step is to learn about your pain. If you understand why you are feeling pain, and are aware of the likelihood of your recovering, you will handle the situation far more positively than someone who does not understand the processes, and whose pain is amplified by his or her fear, foreboding and feelings of helplessness.

Having worked as an osteopathic practitioner in private, as well as state-funded, practices in the United Kingdom, and also in south-east Europe, I have been fascinated to observe the differences in patients' coping skills, both within and between these settings. Much of my work has been with people who are in considerable and often permanent pain, suffering from conditions such as arthritis and fibromyalgia. One clear impression I have gained, supported by medical research, is that learning

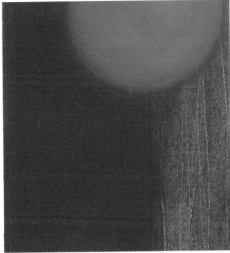

about his or her own condition often helps the person in pain as much as any treatment. Knowledge is power, and understanding your pain gives you power over it.

One of my motivations in writing this book was to bring to a wider audience as much information as possible about pain, based on recent research, and to show what we can do to help ourselves to recover from pain, or to cope with it. The sheer range of causes, types and intensities of pain, and of ways in which it can be modified, blocked, eased or eliminated, is beyond the scope of any one book. What can be done here is to convey the essence of the pain story, giving you the knowledge that will empower you to deal with your inevitable periods of pain most appropriately. Instead of "no pain, no gain", this book aims to give you "more information, less pain".

Leon Chaitow

chapter one

UNDERSTANDING YOUR PAIN

Of all symptoms pain is the one that is most likely to drive us to consult our doctor. While there are a great many ways of easing or "killing" pain, using conventional and alternative methods, we should always try to understand what is causing the pain before attempting to eliminate it. When a fire alarm rings, finding the source of the fire is far more urgent than switching off the alarm.

In this chapter we embark on our journey of discovery into the nature of pain – what causes it, what it signifies and how it operates. Along the way we will explore the powerful connection between mind and body, and the remarkable processes of self-repair, which are constantly at work keeping us in the best condition possible. How and why pain develops, and whether it should be seen as something to deal with ourselves, something to get help for, something to learn from, or (at times) something to ignore, are all part of this journey.

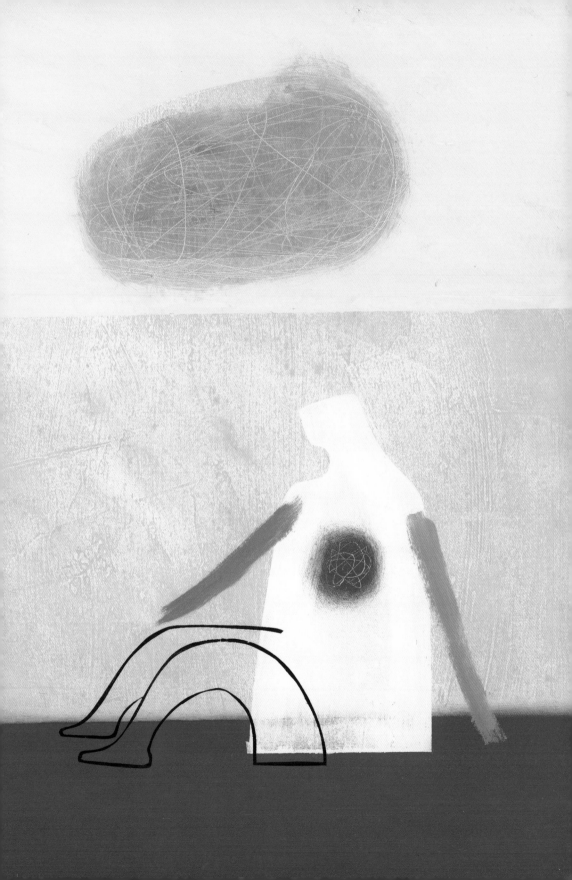

WHAT IS PAIN?

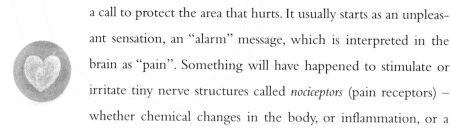

Initially, pain serves as a message of distress, danger or damage – a call to protect the area that hurts. It usually starts as an unpleasant sensation, an "alarm" message, which is interpreted in the brain as "pain". Something will have happened to stimulate or irritate tiny nerve structures called *nociceptors* (pain receptors) – whether chemical changes in the body, or inflammation, or a purely mechanical cause, such as pressure, stretching or tearing.

The body never lies.

Martha Graham
(1894–1991)

Nociceptors are uncovered nerve endings that exist in most tissues of the body, in greater numbers where we are most sensitive. Each nociceptor has a threshold that has to be exceeded before it reports to the brain (via nerves) that there is a problem. This threshold varies from situation to situation, and from person to person, so that what would feel like a minor discomfort for one person may be sensed as severe pain for another.

Although the alarm messages that we perceive as pain usually (but not always) start in the part that hurts, this is not where we actually feel pain. Instead, pain is felt in the brain, by means of the virtual body map that resides there – if this seems strange, consider that many amputees continue to feel "phantom" pain in the missing limb long after it has been removed.

And just to make matters a little more complicated, consider that some pain does not even originate from where we feel the hurt. Pain messages arising from local areas in the muscles and traveling along nerves toward the spine and from there to the brain can be re-routed, so that the pain is felt somewhere else altogether. This is known as reflex, or referred, pain (see also pp.20–21) – one of the commonest examples of which is angina pain felt in the left arm (and other areas) but deriving from distress in the heart muscles.

Pain can be described as acute or chronic. Acute pain derives from a condition that builds rapidly to a crisis, such as a sprained ankle, whereas chronic pain is longer-lasting, more deep-seated

MEASURING YOUR PAIN

Pain is a personal experience – as difficult to measure and express objectively as hunger or thirst, happiness or sadness. You cannot say exactly how much a pain hurts, only that it is, for example, mild, moderate, severe or agonizing. However, your idea of what constitutes an "agonizing pain" may be very different from someone else's.

You can use the calibrated line shown below as a template to incorporate in a "pain diary" – a journal in which you record aspects of your pain experience (see pp.32–5). By marking your pain level on such a scale each day, you can keep a check on how your pain is changing over time, perhaps in response to different treatments.

MARK THE LINE AT THE LEVEL OF PAIN YOU FEEL RIGHT NOW:
0 = no pain; 3 = mild pain; 5 = moderate, bearable pain;
7 = severe but tolerable pain; 10 = agonizing, unbearable pain

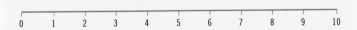

0   1   2   3   4   5   6   7   8   9   10

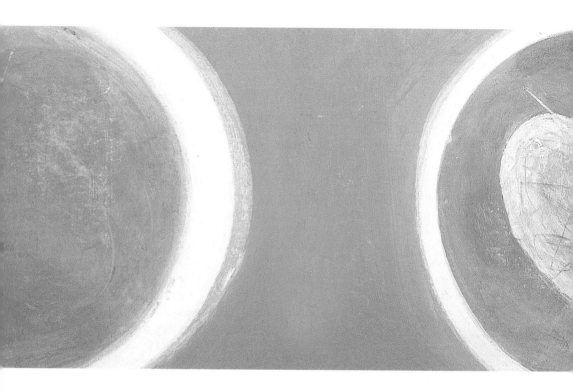

– for example, back pain resulting from poor posture over a long period. The way we experience chronic pain is affected not merely by the physical processes that have caused it, but also by our intellectual and emotional reaction to it. Much depends on the "meaning" that we give the pain, which we tend to process through our individual experiences and expectations. Take, again, the arm pain of angina, which is similar to arm pain originating from hypersensitive points in the muscles of the front of the neck (the *scalenes*). Your attitude toward the pain would be very different if you thought it were a neck-muscle problem rather than a heart problem! What pain means to us, and the circumstances out of which it emerges, can radically affect its perceived potency. If we understand the cause of our pain, we are more likely to react to it in a constructive way.

Pain is sometimes positively useful. If you burn, graze, cut or bruise your arm, you know why it hurts afterwards. Days later such an injured area may still be red and painful owing to the inflammatory process, without which the tissues could not heal (see pp.28–9). These healing tissues need to be treated with care so that they remodel themselves properly – the continued hurt is a warning to avoid doing too much too soon.

Sometimes, however, the cause of a pain is anything but clear, calling for expert investigation. In some cases the original cause of pain may be long gone, but its effects live on in the form of a constant discomfort or worse. This occurs in conditions such as shingles (herpes zoster), after which left-over burning pain can continue for many years, serving no warning purpose at all. If you don't know why something is hurting, you need to find out.

So, there are a number of interconnected elements, which we need to explore before we can learn how to handle pain effectively. There are the nociceptors – what causes their thresholds to be breached and how they signal to the brain; there is the reception of pain messages in the brain; and, most importantly, there is your interpretation of these messages. Understanding these stages in the pain experience will allow you to face pain more positively and to control it more successfully.

THE PAIN EXPERIENCE

There is often a huge emotional content to pain outside of its signal-and-response nature. This content – frequently derived from unfounded and unnecessary fear – produces many signals, other than those related directly to the pain, and these signals need to be interpreted by the brain. In order to understand how pain works, and therefore how we can control it, we need to consider both its mechanics and its psychological overtones.

Numerous tests have shown that people can usually learn to cope with even severe pain if challenged to do so, or if the circumstances in which the pain occurs demand that they ignore it. For example, we are much more tolerant of productive pain (such as that associated with childbirth or life-enhancing surgery) than pain deriving from an accident. If we have difficulty coming to terms with our pain, we risk falling into the trap of "pain behaviour" (see also box, p.43). Pain behaviour involves over-compensating for a painful condition by avoiding performing everyday tasks, such as getting dressed or preparing meals, or by performing them more slowly, and with a greater sense of trepidation, than necessary.

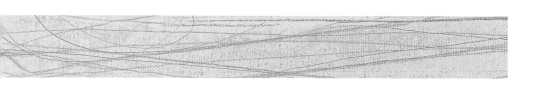

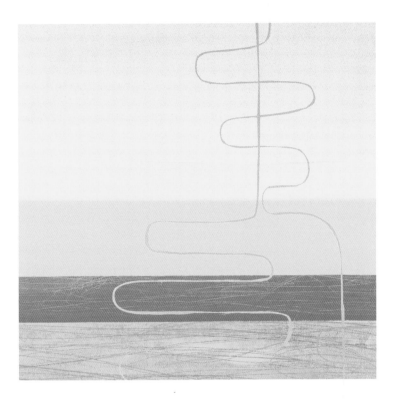

Another factor that seems to influence how we respond to pain, even at extreme levels, is our cultural background. Research has demonstrated that people from different cultures can respond to the same amount of pain in very different ways.

Work by Drs Ronald Melzack and Patrick D. Wall – perhaps the world's leading pain researchers – shows that when painful electric shocks are given to sensitive areas of the body, the level at which they are reported as "intolerable" varies widely depending on the cultural background of the volunteers being tested. For example, in one of their studies, Nepalese volunteers reported severe pain only when receiving a far higher level of electrical stimulation than European volunteers.

In another experiment, Melzack and Wall demonstrated that people could be challenged to increase their tolerance of the pain caused by holding their hand in icy water if they were told that another person had been able to keep their hand in the water for longer than they had. This type of research suggests

SHUTTING THE PAIN GATE

Gentle rubbing, touching or pressing of an area of the body produces messages that are transmitted toward the brain along different nerve pathways from those used to transmit pain messages. These milder sensations derive from the stimulation of very low-threshold nerve endings, which are far more easily activated than pain receptors. What's more, mild-sensation messages travel more quickly and there-fore reach the brain sooner than pain messages. This means that you can partially block the pain signals coming from a painful area by stimulating it gently – we call this "shutting the pain gate".

Awareness of the "pain gate" and how to close it (even if only partially) has led to the widespread practice of numerous therapies. These include: manual pressure techniques, such as acupressure and shiatsu; acupuncture (both plain and electrical); and massage. TENS (transcutaneous electrical nerve stimulation) machines also have a pain-blocking effect – they work by passing a very mild electrical current across painful regions. Not only do these therapies "shut the pain gate", but they also induce the body to release natural painkilling hormones (endorphins and enkephalins).

that we possess a built-in ability to alter our pain tolerance through the power of suggestion, which in turn has important implications for how we can improve our handling of pain.

Research also suggests that our gender and "personality type" can have a bearing on the way in which we deal with painful conditions. Women handle pain better, but consult a physician about it more readily, than men do; as we might expect, laid-back, calm people seem far better able to cope with quite severe pain, compared with those who are highly nervous and anxious.

There is, therefore, an accumulation of evidence relating to "mind control" over pain. By observing the varying ways in which different people experience similar types of pain, researchers have been able to develop tactics to help all people – not just those about to give birth, or from Nepal – to manage their pain better and sometimes even to overcome it completely. A science, known as Cognitive Behavioural Therapy, has grown out of this research and this forms a major part of the work of dedicated pain clinics.

Managing pain means being able to find ways of living with it so that it does not dominate everyday activities, or prevent a fulfilling and active life. Many of these strategies will be discussed in more detail in later sections of this book. They include relaxation and meditation methods (see chapter three, pp.50–75), hydrotherapy (see pp.104–7), and techniques that put the "gate theory" of pain into practice (see box, opposite).

TRACING PAIN

It's not always easy to know where pain is coming from. Sometimes it's pretty obvious – if, say, you stub your toe or bump your head. But often the pain you feel in one place originates somewhere else. This is because the "wiring" of the body is extremely complex – despite hundreds of years of research we still only partially understand it.

In order to make sense of the nervous system we first have to classify it into different sub-systems. The autonomic nervous system, which governs those aspects of the body over which we have little or no conscious control, is itself divided into the sympathetic and the parasympathetic nervous systems, which respectively stimulate or moderate functions such as the rate at which you breathe, or your heart beats. Within these systems and sub-systems a host of "reflex pathways" exist which help in the management of the astonishingly intricate functioning of the human organism. It is along these pathways that messages such as pain are referred from one area to another. For example, viscero-somatic pathways carry pain that originates in an organ to a more mechanical part of the body, such as angina pain felt in the arm. Pain traveling in the opposite direction (along a somatico-visceral pathway) includes that felt in the heart, but caused by irritated nerve structures in the pectoral muscles. Messages can also be transmitted from one movable part of the body to another (along a somatico-somatic pathway). A simple example of this is the defensive reflex that tells your arm to move your hand away when you touch something hot.

Pain felt in a part of the body may even have an emotional, rather than a physical, cause. An example of this psycho-somatic pain is the stomach ache you might feel before an exam.

In some cases, a single event can give rise to more than one pain message traveling along more than one pathway. For example, if you were to fall and twist your back, the vertebra that you twisted would itself be painful afterwards, but you might also suffer pain in one of your legs. There could be many possible explanations for the referred leg pain: the vertebra might be pressing onto a nerve; or you might have irritated some nerve structures in the joints connecting the vertebrae to each other; or you may have altered your posture to compensate for the pain in your back, thereby triggering pain in your leg ... or it could be something else altogether. The wonderful aspect of all this confusion is that when researchers compare the progress of different back injuries of this sort they find that, with or without treatment or medication, most are better within four weeks. The body heals itself, and when it cannot, treatment is needed.

THE STRESS EFFECT

Stress is often thought of as a condition that affects only the mind. However, in its broadest sense, stress can be defined as any internal or external factor that demands that your mind or body adapt in some way. Because it can lead to or aggravate many forms of pain, we need to understand how stress operates.

Stress factors are grouped into three main categories: biochemical (for example, dietary imbalances, infection, allergies and environmental toxicity); biomechanical (over- or underuse of the body, and poor posture and injuries); and psychosocial (emotional pressures, anxiety, fear, depression, and so on). Combinations of these factors are affecting all of us much of the time. Not everyone is able to cope with the same amount of stress – the way we each handle the pressures of life depends on our inborn characteristics and the acquired patterns of response

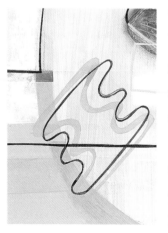

we have developed through our past experience. When we reach our stress threshold, the self-repair processes of our mind and body stop adapting adequately to the multiple stresses, like a strip of elastic that has been stretched too far and for too long.

However, stress can be the by-product of positive, healthy changes to your lifestyle. Let's say that you take up fitness training. The first few sessions lead to stiffness and muscle soreness, but if you sustain your exercise routine your body will adapt to the bio-mechanical stress by building new muscle fibres, and improving your circulation to meet the new demand for oxygen.

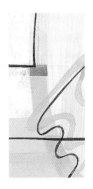

More often, though, stress results from sustained inappropri-ate activity. If you sit slumped at a desk working a computer (or you play the guitar, dig the garden or drive a car) for too long, your body adapts to these stress demands by tightening up the overused muscles, and soon stiffness, and later pain, develop. (This is another form of biomechanical stress and is often known as repetitive strain injury – see p.142.)

So far our examples have related to biomechanical stress, but what happens when the stresses are multiple? Take, for example, someone whose work and leisure pastimes have helped to cre-ate a physically and psychologically stressful lifestyle – insuffi-cient rest time, inability to ease up, time pressures, repetitive or posturally uncomfortable activities, inadequate exercise levels. Add emotional issues, owing to work, education, relationship or economic factors, with sleep-pattern disturbances and a diet that is less than ideal, and an alarming picture emerges. Each of the stress factors may be insufficient to produce a problem on its own, but when combined they can set the scene for pain and other adverse symptoms to develop. These symptoms then pro-duce more stress as they, in turn, force the body to adapt. The good news is that just as a watch can be water proofed, so a person can – to a very large extent – be "stress proofed".

HELP YOUR BODY TO HELP ITSELF

The body has a built-in repair potential – an automatic inclination to restore its natural equilibrium (otherwise known as homeostasis). Normally, wounds heal, broken bones mend and infections clear. However, the efficiency with which homeostatic mechanisms can do their work depends on your unique characteristics, both the ones you were born with and those you acquire through life, such as nutritional habits and posture.

SOME OF THE MULTIPLE
STRESSES OF LIFE

- Nutritional deficiencies
- Allergies, infections, inflammation
- Exposure to toxicity
- Abuse of drugs, nicotine, alcohol

- Acquired traits, e.g. previous
  and current ailments
- Personal hygiene
- Exercise and sleep factors

- Attention to hygiene, exercise,
  rest or sleep

- Unique genetic traits
- Learned behaviour

- Awareness of general
  health-maintenance issues

The "staircase" below shows how life's multiple stresses can mount up to overload your defence and repair systems, which leads to a situation known as heterostasis. When this happens we generally need outside help to restore homeostasis. We call that outside agency "treatment".

Our self-healing capability is enormous, and it is vital that we do not lose sight of this great gift. Our task when we are ill, or in pain, is to attempt to remove obstacles to recovery, to support as best we can the multiple functions that make up homeostasis, and to avoid interfering with self-healing processes.

The "staircase" below shows the stresses that can escalate to overwhelm you. However, under the stairs are treatments to counter each of these stresses.

- Poor posture
- Over- and misuse of body
- Injuries, surgery
- Degenerative joint problems

- Exercise, stretching, Pilates, yoga, t'ai chi, physiotherapy, massage, osteopathy, acupuncture

- Stress levels (interpersonal, at work, financial)
- Anxiety, depression, anger
- Isolation, poor self-image

- Stress management, counseling, psychotherapy
- Breathing retraining, relaxation methods (eg. meditation, visualization, autogenic training)
- Spiritual renewal, social support

- Reformed dietary habits, appropriate supplements, herbs, homeopathy, detox programs
- Attention to possible pollutants at home and work

SOME OF THE TREATMENT AND SELF-HELP OPTIONS THAT CAN AID RECOVERY

TOLERANCE LEVELS

At times, parts of our body, perhaps through overuse, are subjected to sustained stress. In these cases the nociceptors can become sensitized, leading to one of two very different results.

When the volume on a radio or TV is set too low, our brains interpret voices as background noise – we are unable to understand what is actually being said. In the same way, there is a threshold of stimulation below which nociceptors do not report pain to the brain.

If the prolonged irritation of the pain receptors is mild to moderate, a process known as habituation takes place. The reporting of pain to the brain actually diminishes. This response suggests that the brain and nervous system can recognize when messages are unimportant. One of our objectives in managing chronic, "useless" pain situations is to achieve habituation, so that the brain can ignore the pain messages.

Precisely the opposite effect can arise in response to intense, rapidly repeating pain stimuli, such as those produced by a diseased organ – say, the heart or kidneys. The nerves that carry pain messages from the affected organ can become "facilitated" – that is to say, more readily irritated. Facilitation, also known as "wind-up", means that pain messages are sent to the brain at very much lower levels of stimulus than if the pain receptors were unfacilitated, or not "wound-up".

Another aspect of "wind-up" is that the facilitated pain receptors start to send signals of pain and distress to the brain, not only when directly stimulated, but also when other forms of stress affect the mind and body as a whole – for example, in response to any physical effort or to an emotional upset. The

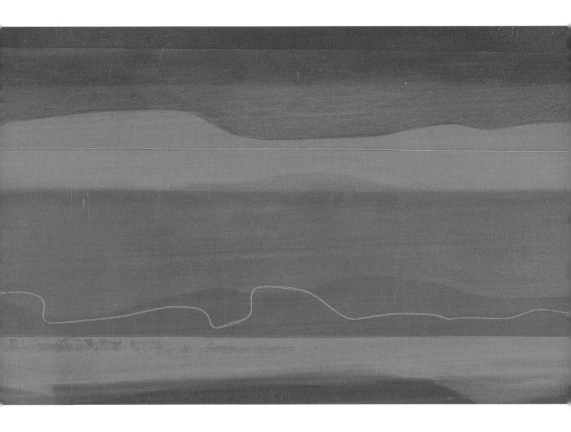

inevitable result of all these stresses being focused on one part of the body is added strain on the facilitated area, which only serves to aggravate the original problem.

What we can learn from these two important features of pain is that the amount of pain we feel and how well we tolerate it depend to a large extent on the way the brain interprets pain messages. Whatever else we do about the pain and its direct causes, clearly we also need to try to reduce our overall stress levels, as these can have considerable influence on the pain load.

INFLAMMATION IS GOOD FOR YOU

Although often painful, inflammation is a natural, and vitally important, tissue-repair mechanism, and helps the body to defend against damage, irritation and infection.

Our defence and repair mechanisms follow remarkable daily rhythms. Those body systems that defend against attack by bacteria or viruses are far more active between roughly ten in the morning and ten in the evening, leaving the night shift for tissue-repair processes, including inflammation. This explains why inflammation is normally worse at night. Stressful events seem to alter these rhythms, so that the inflammatory phase can stay "switched on" during the day. When this happens the defensive phase of the cycle is relatively weakened, leaving the body vulnerable to infection.

Over-the-counter, anti-inflammatory medicines, such as aspirin, should be treated with care, both because of their many potential side-effects (ranging from stomach bleeding to severe liver and kidney problems) and because they are often *too* effective in controlling inflammation. This slows down the repair of damaged tissues, and can cause the patient to use the area too soon and too much, creating even bigger problems.

However, there are many safe, natural methods for easing painful inflammation.

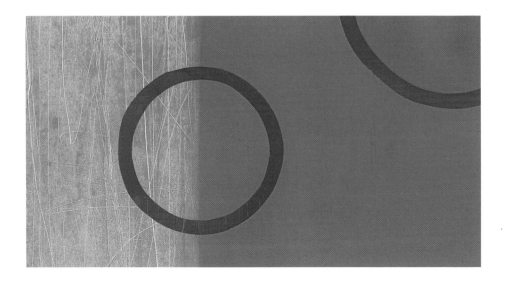

We can gently reduce inflammation (and the related pain) with dietary strategies that cut down our intake of animal fats and increase our intake of fish oils. Animal fats contain large amounts of *arachidonic acid*, from which pro-inflammatory substances in your body, known as *cytokines*, are derived; whereas oily fish, such as sardines, salmon and tuna, contain high levels of *eicosapentenoic acid* (EPA), which studies have shown to counteract inflammatory activity (see also pp.114–15).

Moderating our stress levels can also help. We have seen that stress can interfere with defence-and-repair rhythms – by reducing stress we can reset the body's daily pattern. In addition, high levels of cortisol – the "stress hormone" – are linked to the release of cytokines. Reduced stress leads to reduced cortisol, and therefore moderation of these inflammatory chemicals.

THE PATH TO RECOVERY

The good news is that there are many ways in which we can manage almost all types of pain, and the conditions that cause them. Some of these management techniques can be self-applied, others require treatment administered by conventional or complementary healthcare providers. At this point it is important to emphasize, and re-emphasize, that no pain should be ignored or masked with painkillers (see box, opposite) without first understanding its cause. Remember also that your path to recovery begins with *appropriate* treatment – treatment that is safe and that works with the body's self-repair mechanisms (see pp.24–5), not against them.

Try not to expect too much. Self-repair is not always possible – for example, in cases where pain is caused by chronic, degenerative conditions, such as osteoarthritis. In severe cases, methods used to control pain may need to be extreme: drugs that carry side-effects, or surgery. However, even in such situations the general principles and specific therapies presented in this book can make life more tolerable.

Probably the most important factor governing how fast you travel the path toward recovery is your attitude and the way you make use of your inner reserve of strength – a store that we all have within us. Try to

OVER-THE-COUNTER PAINKILLERS

Many orthodox Western medical methods set out to attack symptoms. If it hurts "kill the pain", and if it's inflamed deactivate the inflammation (see pp.28–9). To be fair, most doctors recognize that this sort of approach is not ideal, as pain (sometimes) and inflammation (almost always) serve key roles in the body's defence and self-repair processes. A failure by patients to appreciate the dangers of unprescribed medication, constant promotion by pharmaceutical companies, and ready availability of medicines without prescription from pharmacies and supermarkets, keep painkilling and anti-inflammatory medication sales booming.

This is not to deny that at times such medication may be a useful first aid. But there are significant dangers in stopping the pain before its message has been understood. For example, a painful knee may signal the onset of an easily managed cartilage problem. However, if the sufferer takes painkillers, then uses the knee in running, jumping or even walking, the damage will worsen – sometimes irreparably. Kill the pain and this is the likely outcome. Recognize the cause and the problem can usually be fixed – and the pain will go away.

One of the first duties of the physician is to educate the masses not to take medicine.

William Osler
(1849–1919)

think constructively about your pain and be proactive in the recovery process. Tackling the management of your pain in a positive way will encourage you to take control of all aspects of your life. Your painful ordeal can provide an opportunity for reflection and change, enabling you to transform your lifestyle in ways you may often have considered, but never had the impetus to follow through.

KEEPING A PAIN DIARY

Can you recall how you felt at any given moment over the past week, and what you had to eat for each meal, and make connections between these factors and the degree of pain you experienced on each day? Most people find it difficult to recall the minutiae of their everyday life, and yet these details probably contain valuable information relating to the pattern and possible causes of your pain symptoms. As no one can realistically be expected to remember everything they do each day, it might be useful to record the information in a diary or on a chart. When

In this sample entry from a pain diary, the intensity of the pain is recorded on a "pain bar". A body map enables you to plot the pain's location or locations. By drawing several concentric circles on the map around the painful area, you can indicate the severity of the pain.

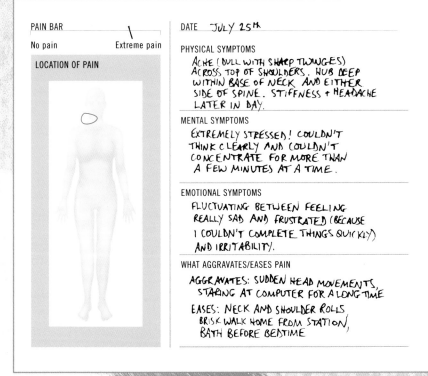

PAIN BAR

No pain   Extreme pain

LOCATION OF PAIN

DATE JULY 25ᵗʰ

PHYSICAL SYMPTOMS
ACHE (DULL WITH SHARP TWINGES) ACROSS TOP OF SHOULDERS. HUB DEEP WITHIN BASE OF NECK AND EITHER SIDE OF SPINE. STIFFNESS + HEADACHE LATER IN DAY.

MENTAL SYMPTOMS
EXTREMELY STRESSED! COULDN'T THINK CLEARLY AND COULDN'T CONCENTRATE FOR MORE THAN A FEW MINUTES AT A TIME.

EMOTIONAL SYMPTOMS
FLUCTUATING BETWEEN FEELING REALLY SAD AND FRUSTRATED (BECAUSE I COULDN'T COMPLETE THINGS QUICKLY) AND IRRITABILITY.

WHAT AGGRAVATES/EASES PAIN
AGGRAVATES: SUDDEN HEAD MOVEMENTS, STARING AT COMPUTER FOR A LONG TIME
EASES: NECK AND SHOULDER ROLLS, BRISK WALK HOME FROM STATION, BATH BEFORE BEDTIME

analyzed by you or a healthcare professional, these records may bring insights to light from apparently unrelated factors.

Use the sample diary entry below, and the list of questions on the following page, as a basis for your own journal tailored to your particular requirements. Writing down this information gives you a chance to sort out a jumble of facts – things that you already know but have not had time to organize to useful effect. As you make regular entries in your diary, you may well notice patterns emerging in your daily activities and your symptoms. By altering aspects of your daily life to take account of any correlations, you can manage your experience of pain.

PLAN	ACTUAL
DIET DRINK: 2 LITRES WATER + EAT 4 PIECES FRUIT BREAKFAST: OATS (SKIMMED MILK) LUNCH: TOMATO SOUP (WITH ROLL - NO BUTTER) DINNER: CHICKEN + SALAD	ALL DONE! (EXCEPT ONE SNACK ON A BISCUIT BAR AT MID-AFTERNOON)
MOVEMENT A.M.: 10 MINS NECK ROLLS + SHOULDER ROLLS P.M.: 10 MINS BICEP STRETCHES + BACK STRETCHES + HEAD + NECK ROLLS	ALL DONE!
RELAXATION 10 MINUTE VISUALIZED MEDITATION BEFORE BED 5 MINUTES BREATHING (ANYTIME)	MISSED THE BREATHING - SCHEDULE IN MORE FIRMLY FOR TOMORROW
GOALS ∗ LEAVE WORK ON TIME (TO INCREASE RELAXATION TIME) ∗ CALL A FRIEND (TO KEEP IN TOUCH)	LEFT 15 MINUTES LATE - AN IMPROVEMENT CALLED ANNE - IT WAS GREAT TO TALK TO HER. SHE'S DOING REALLY WELL!

Use your diary to set yourself manageable daily targets for improved diet, flexibility and relaxation. Establishing general lifestyle goals will help you gain control over your life – and your pain. Make a separate column to record how successful you have been in achieving your aims.

QUESTIONS YOU CAN USE TO STRUCTURE YOUR PAIN DIARY:

• Is the pain constant or intermittent? If the latter, what pattern does it follow? After what activities does it hurt?

• What sort of pain is it? (Aching, burning, sharp, stabbing, cramp-like, tingling, and so on.)

• Is there swelling, redness or heat in the area of pain?

• Does it still hurt when you rest, or does rest ease the pain?

• Is it easier when you move around? If so, what sort of movement eases it (slow stretching, walking, and so on)?

• Is the pain affected by certain foods and drinks? If so, which?

• Is the pain affected by emotional factors? If so, which?

• If you are female, is the pain affected for better or worse by aspects of your menstrual cycle?

A diary (or part of it) can be specifically focused. For example, if there seems to be a link between a chronic pain and certain foods, you might find it useful to keep a "symptom score sheet" (see example, opposite) combined with a food diary to assess the effects of the inclusion or exclusion of particular foods on your pain pattern (see pp.120–24). List everything you ate, as well as the times of day you had your meals. Record any variation in the pattern of your symptoms. Try to note down the precise time at which the symptoms varied.

Your diary should give you room to describe not just your physical symptoms but also your feelings in relation to your pain (as well as to life events) to see how they might be influencing each other. If you feel anger, fear, anxiety or any other strong emotions, notes in the diary offer a chance to explore these matters, perhaps with the help of someone else.

While you should be careful to record information accurately in the diary, as regularly as you can, it is important not to become obsessive about it. See it as a record, something to aid your memory, which can help you to understand the bigger picture surrounding your pain.

In the score sheet below, stress at work seems to make neck, head and fatigue symptoms worse; Pilates exercise, rest and massage seem to have a beneficial effect on overall pain scores.

SYMPTOM SCORE SHEET						
DATE	MAY 12th	MAY 13th	MAY 14th	MAY 15th	MAY 16th	MAY 17th
NECK PAIN	2	1	1	2	3	2
HEADACHE	2	1	1	3	3	2
FATIGUE	3	2	1	3	2	1
INDIGESTION	1	0	0	2	1	0
SLEEP	1	2	0	2	1	1
CONCENTRATION	2	3	1	2	1	1
TOTAL	11	9	4	14	11	7
notes	STARTED PILATES CLASS	ACHED AFTER PILATES, BUT FELT LOOSER	GOOD PAIN DAY! CHINESE MEAL	STRESSFUL DAY AT WORK	NO DESK WORK TODAY. RESTED	PILATES CLASS + MASSAGE

Every day at the same time of the day score each symptom for the previous 24 hours:
3 = worst possible; 2 = moderately bad; 1 = mild; 0 = no problem

chapter two

POSITIVE ATTITUDES

Do you see pain as a challenge or as a threat? If you are an instinctively positive person who reflects on life's demands and problems and tries to find solutions to them, you are likely to view pain as a challenge – an obstacle that you can overcome. If, on the other hand, you take the negative approach, seeing stressful life events as being largely beyond your influence, you will probably view pain as a threat – something terrible for which there is no remedy other than stoical endurance.

"Hardiness" is a term used in psychology to describe a group of traits that, when they are present in a person's way of coping with life, make for more positive approaches and outcomes. The good news is that it is possible to develop hardiness traits, and to see favourable results emerging from even the darkest situations. This chapter explores these opportunities.

TURNING THE MENTAL KEY

The so-called "hardiness factor", which has been identified as a positive, helpful, life-enhancing characteristic – invaluable in facing up to painful conditions – calls for the presence of three main attributes.

The first, and most crucial, of these is a sense of **control**, a recognition that you are capable of influencing life's events for the better. Many people who experience pain (and even those who don't) have feelings of powerlessness, of being at the mercy of fate. When you begin to exercise control over any part of your life – and in this context that means over aspects of your pain – you take the first step toward empowerment. Even if the control you exercise over your pain is only temporary and partial – perhaps something as simple as booking an acupuncture session or taking up yoga – the encouragement you will derive from this breakthrough will spur you on to dominate a condition that previously seemed to be dominating you.

The only way to do something is to do it.

Laurence Olivier (1907–89)

The second main hardiness feature is **commitment** – a commitment to involve oneself in society and the lives of others. Pain can make it all too easy to withdraw from other people, to avoid social contact, to become isolated. But to a large extent this is a choice we make for ourselves, and like all choices it means there are other possible options, too. The media is constantly presenting examples of individuals who have suffered

UNLOCK YOUR POTENTIAL

There is no shortcut to exercising control, to reducing your sense of isolation, or to viewing problems as challenges rather than threats. This exercise will help you take the first steps – the most important and most difficult – toward strengthening those aspects of hardiness that are not features of your personality already. As you find yourself becoming more and more confident in these 3 techniques, you will find that they become second nature, and without your even realizing, they will influence your way of approaching all aspects of your life.

1. To foster a sense of control, identify a treatment or therapy that is likely to help you. Write a list of steps that you need to take – say, making appointments or buying equipment – to make your project take shape. Set yourself target dates for each step. Writing down your plan will give you a tangible starting point, rather than just a mass of good intentions in your head.

2. To avoid cutting yourself off from the outside world, call a friend once a week. Make sure that you don't talk just about your pain, but also discuss what is happening to them. Arrange to meet them when you feel ready – but don't rush yourself.

3. To help you view obstacles as challenges, transform your negative statements into positive ones. Train yourself to stop in your tracks when you find yourself saying something like, "I don't stand a chance". Revise your statement and say it aloud – for example, "Although it may be difficult, I can do it".

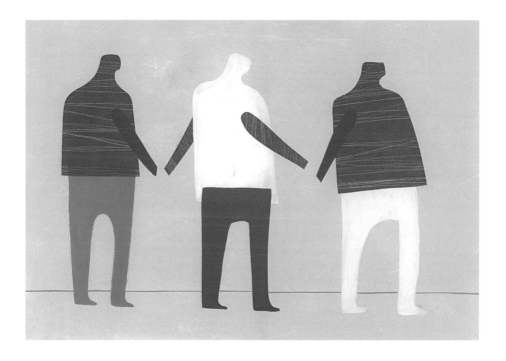

enormously, and yet who have overcome the vicissitudes of their lives to become beacons of hope, examples to us all. People who, despite being crippled by injury or born with major disabilities, have set aside their scars and pain and made a positive contribution to society. Some such individuals may have inborn personality traits that help them toward this degree of commitment, but they are also choosing to exercise these traits, refusing to be beaten by circumstances. Research shows that commitment is greatly helped by a social support system, whether this involves friends, family, a partner or professional advisers. Even if you feel that you are alone, there are always people to whom you can turn. Choosing to ignore those who can offer support can add to feelings of isolation.

There are a number of ways – some obvious, others less so – in which you can engage with the people around you. At the simplest end of the scale try speaking to someone frankly, uncomplainingly about your pain, so that they (and you) come to a clearer understanding of your problems. Or you could join a local self-help group, where people in a similar situation to you meet to support each other and discuss issues relating to their shared condition. Another option might be to identify someone in need and to do what *you* can to help *them*. In this way you will not only benefit the person you are helping, but also force yourself to look beyond your own suffering.

The third characteristic of hardiness is a sense of **challenge** – for example, the ability to see an illness not as a calamity, but as an opportunity to test yourself and to emerge stronger. This is perhaps the most difficult hardiness element to acquire, especially if previously you have tended toward cynicism or pessimism. Changing your frame of mind so that the world becomes a place of challenges, somewhere in which certain things have to be overcome, may seem impossible – but it isn't. Research has suggested that by making a conscious effort to view life more optimistically, your expectations and behaviour will change accordingly, resulting in more positive outcomes than you had previously imagined possible.

MIND OVER MATTER

Under hypnosis, someone who has been handed an ice cube and told that it is intensely hot will feel burning and drop it. They may even develop a blister in response to the "heat" of the ice cube! The mind controls what we feel, as well as the response, and if it is persuaded that there is danger (even when, in reality, there is none) it will defend the body in a way it deems appropriate. Conversely, people who suffer injuries such as broken limbs or torn muscles in battle or in intense sporting situations often feel no pain at the time. They disassociate themselves from the pain – it becomes unimportant.

If it is possible for the mind to delete pain, or to modify it, it should also be possible to find ways of learning how to apply such techniques consciously, and so to exercise the benefits of mind control in the management of pain.

Hypnotherapy is one such technique that can help you change the way you perceive your pain (others include biofeedback, see p.53, and visualization, see pp.68–9). A qualified hypnotherapist will work with you to construct a "script" that will modify any of your beliefs and feelings that are hampering you. (As a first step, you may be encouraged to rename your pain as "discomfort".) Having guided you into a state of deep relaxation, the therapist will recite the script to you. It might include something like the following: "See your discomfort – it has a size and a shape. Watch it change shape, get smaller, lighter. Feel its effect on you getting less and less". In time, you can record the script onto audio cassette and practise self-hypnosis.

PAIN BEHAVIOUR

The power of the mind is so strong that it can have one drawback. If you *believe* that the pain in your body represents a threat to life itself, or that it is likely to result in serious disability, you will tend to behave in a way that protects you from feeling the pain, which will probably prevent you from functioning normally. Being careful, avoiding aggravation of the condition or the pain, is one thing, but it is quite another to become ultra-cautious – to allow what is known as "pain behaviour" to dominate your life. If you avoid everyday activities "just in case" they upset the painful condition, it may be that your belief in the pain is greater than your belief in the possibility of recovery. There are two ways to modify this negative approach:

• **Alter your attitude** – learn more about your condition, and see that it may actually be made worse by inactivity (see pp.92–5).

• **Alter your behaviour** – become active in the self-management of your pain, your emotions and your environment, and develop a structured plan to gradually increase your levels of activity, with broadening horizons rather than shrinking ones.

To get back on the road to "wellness behaviour", try making a list of pleasurable activities that you now avoid doing because of your pain. Think about which ones it may be possible to take up again and write down how you are going to achieve your aims. Make a start on at least one item within the next 24 hours.

Nothing has any power over me, other than that which I give it through my conscious thoughts.

Anthony Robbins (1960–)

AFFIRMATIONS

When pain is severe, prolonged feelings of helplessness can be overwhelming. Used with faith in their effectiveness, affirmations – repeated positive statements – can bolster our determination to overcome the enslavement of pain.

The pairs of statements shown below are just examples, on which you may or may not choose to base your own affirmations. When constructing your own statements ensure that you do not use any negative or hesitant language. For example, "I can achieve any ambition I set my mind to. I am positive and assured" is far more positive than "I might be able to achieve my

When pain makes you anxious and tense

My body and mind bathe in the light of the spirit.

I let go of my worries. I am free to reach my goals.

When pain brings depression

My pain is a fraction of my life. My fulfilment is infinitely larger.

My life is still under my control. My self, and my relationships, are whole.

When pain returns

The body follows its own wisdom. Healing continues.

Even summer skies have clouds. I have come through before.

ambitions if I try. I am not negative or lacking assurance".

A key word in deciding to use affirmations is "choice". Choosing to listen to the advice of those who advocate affirmation tactics is, in itself, affirmative action. Of course, to have doubts about the validity of such claims is perfectly understandable. However, when you need to create a positive sense of purpose in the face of a painful condition, scepticism about using a process that can patently do no harm, and that might help, is self-limiting. Put aside your reservations and approach affirmations as though they were unquestionably valuable. Try them regularly, as often as you can, especially when you are feeling down. Treat it as your goal to prove that they work.

When pain makes you irritable

No one is responsible for my pain. I will reach out to everyone I value.

I am a calm pool, endlessly fed by the love of family and friends.

When pain makes you feel isolated

Others hold me in their love, even when they are absent.

My contribution is undiminished, even when I need to rest.

When pain requires great strength

I have the will to defeat my pain, to live as fully as I can.

I can achieve any ambition I set my mind to. I am positive and assured.

MAKING IT HAPPEN

Good intentions are rarely enough. If you want your plans to become a reality, it is important to set yourself appropriate, attainable targets, to have a clear idea of what you need to do to achieve them, and, above all, to nurture the strong sense of motivation that will spur you on – even through the tough times.

Motivation involves a desire to change things for the better and requires a belief that the changes you are asking yourself to

A journey of a thousand miles must begin with a single step.

Lao-Tzu
(604–531BCE)

PERSONAL RESOURCES

Health psychologists have identified four personality areas, known as our "personal resources", which have a significant impact on how well motivated we are likely to be in applying self-help strategies:

• **Body awareness** *is the ability to focus on different parts of your body in turn and to understand the needs of each – the autogenic training exercise on p.56 will help you to improve your body awareness.*

• **Self-focus** *involves accepting yourself and your needs, being able to take care of yourself, and having a sense of your own value. Visualizations (see pp.68–9) and affirmations (see pp.44–5) can encourage these qualities.*

• **Locus of control** *depends on whether you see events as being out of your control, or whether you believe you can influence them (see p.38). You can learn to move your locus from beyond you to within you.*

• **Coping ability** *involves recognizing your current limitations and working within them. Someone with little coping ability is liable to ignore their pain and overdo things, causing a setback in their recovery.*

make can indeed bring about an improvement. Your belief should be based on realistic objectives, not false hopes, which is why you should gather information, understand the whys and wherefores of whatever changes you are making. Armed with this knowledge, you will be making a conscious choice to take the path to wellness and recovery.

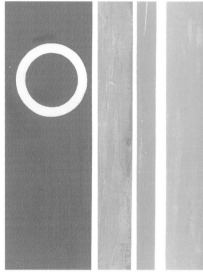

An obvious and appropriate place to start your fact-finding mission is with your doctor (although there is value in finding things out for yourself, from, say, reference books or the internet). Traditionally, the relationship between patient and doctor has been an unequal one – the doctor gives instructions and our trust in the doctor means that we obey without question, and without understanding the reasoning behind the prescribed treatment. However, it may be more constructive to think of the doctor–patient relationship as a partnership, in which the patient actively agrees to a course of action having understood the rationale behind it. Results of studies suggest that the better we understand why we are expected to exercise, or alter our diet, or apply relaxation methods, and so on, the more likely we are to find the motivation to persist with the treatment.

How well do you follow a plan, or take health advice? The truth is that even when we are well and free from pain every single one of us could make a list of things we ought to be doing (or ought to stop doing) that would almost certainly make us healthier, now or in the long run. And there have undoubtedly been times when you have ignored some of the sound, health-enhancing advice given to you by your doctor.

This is human nature – it's worth being aware of it as you start to make plans for recovery from pain, so that you avoid weighing yourself down with blame or guilt when you fail to do everything you set out to accomplish. It's all too easy to give up entirely when you find yourself not quite able or willing to do all that's needed. By anticipating at the outset the possibility of difficult periods, lapses or partial failure, you are less likely to abandon your plan completely.

As we have seen, reducing the mechanical, chemical and psychological stresses on your body will lead to better functioning of your repair and regeneration systems (see pp.24–5). As you see initial improvements in your experience of pain, your motivation should get stronger. Unfortunately, though, the chances are that your motivation will plateau and begin to tail off when you reach a marked reduction in your pain. To ward off the danger of complacency, you may need to freshen up your strategy by regularly re-evaluating your goals and the methods you use to achieve them (see p.155). Reviewing your pain diary on a regular basis will enable you not only to build up an understanding of your condition, to set your goals and monitor your success in achieving them, but also to identify new directions to take.

PROBLEM SOLVING

It is all too easy to slip into the habit of avoiding everyday tasks that your pain makes difficult. This exercise will help you to work out – and to carry out – plans to make these activities more manageable.

1. Write down a list of any tasks that you find awkward because of your pain. These could include getting dressed, cooking, going shopping, or doing something specific at work, such as sitting at a computer.

2. Choose one of your problem areas. Give it a "difficulty score" from 0 to 10, where not being able to do it at all would be worth 10, and being able to do it perfectly and painlessly would be worth 0. What's it "worth" right now?

3. Now, make a list of any tactics, equipment, assistance, training or relearning of skills that might help you to achieve the difficult task.

4. Assess your list of strategies. Which are the easiest things to do? Do them first. Do any of them require outside help? Get it. Are they things you can organize for yourself? Do so. Start to put your plan into action.

5. Repeat steps 2 to 4 for each of the items on your original list of problem areas.

6. Each week score the activities again in your pain diary – watch the totals drop as your plans take shape.

chapter three

FINDING PEACE

Imagine yourself calm and pain free. In the previous chapter you saw how it is possible to use the power of your mind to begin to feel this way. This chapter brings you tried-and-tested methods designed to guide you toward what is known as the "relaxation response". This is the exact opposite of the "stress response" (in which we tense ourselves and withdraw from painful situations).

The ways in which relaxation can be achieved differ from person to person. For some, it might involve physical tensing and releasing of muscles, to "remind" the body what it feels like to let go. For others, breathing or meditation exercises may be more effective. Try a range of the techniques presented in this chapter and practise regularly those that work best for you. By repeated application you should see heartening improvements emerging over the coming weeks.

RELEASE YOUR MUSCLES TO RELEASE YOUR MIND

An inability to relax physically can create a vicious circle of increasing tension, fatigue, anxiety and pain. Fortunately, you can learn techniques that will allow you to recognize and to counteract the effects of physical tension.

When you are in pain, or are anxious, your muscles become tense. Tense muscles require more oxygen than relaxed ones, but the irony is that the blood vessels that carry fresh, oxygenated blood into the muscle are constricted by the tightened tissue, and the blood is prevented from reaching all parts of the muscle. This is particularly likely to happen if the muscle is not being used all that strenuously. Also, when muscles are tense, waste products are prevented from draining out of them efficiently. Poor oxygenation of muscle tissue and retention of metabolic wastes lead to discomfort and stiffness – which tend to create even more tension! Fatigue is also likely, because keeping muscles tense wastes a lot of energy.

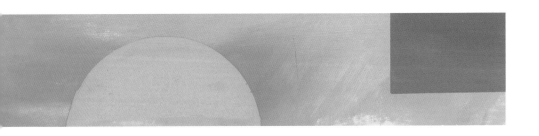

BIOFEEDBACK

Biofeedback enables you to alter aspects of the way your body functions – warming areas, relaxing areas – just by thinking about them. A small, relatively inexpensive device, which you connect to yourself with electrodes, measures an aspect of your body's biological functioning, such as blood pressure, heart rate or brainwaves, and feeds this information back to you in the form of a flashing light or a beep for every, say, heartbeat.

By entering a deeply relaxed state, in which you focus your whole attention on the biofeedback machine, you can train yourself (virtually by trial and error) to increase or reduce the interval between the flashes or beeps, and, by so doing, to alter the body function – for example, to reduce your blood pressure or your heart rate.

It is usually necessary to receive some initial instruction before practising this technique on your own. Biofeedback has a very high success rate in pain relief and is often used and taught by physiotherapists and in specialized pain clinics.

This tense state, known as "sympathetic arousal", is part of the "fight or flight" mechanism, originally intended to prepare you to run away from danger, or to defend yourself against it. When the "alarm" is raised, adrenaline is released, which automatically causes your muscles to tense. At the same time, your heartbeat, breathing rate and blood pressure all increase to service the anticipated demands of the body. Many other instant-reflex events occur – these are all reversed as soon as the danger has passed. However, if danger continues – if there were an extended period of emergency – then your muscles would stay permanently tense, and you would remain constantly prepared for action. This prolonged state of sympathetic arousal is a recipe for exhaustion and pain.

In time, muscle tension can become habitual. This physical unease can feed back to the brain messages that you are anxious or agitated, taking you still further away from a state of relaxation. You may reach a point at which you are no longer even aware how tense your muscles are, and releasing them becomes almost impossible. This means that if you try to relax, the effect will probably be the opposite – you may tighten your muscles even more, because you will have forgotten what relaxation feels like. In such a situation relaxation has to be relearned.

A word of caution is needed here. When someone who has not been able to relax for a long time finally achieves feelings of release, the first experiences of letting go can be almost frightening, as though they are losing control. So be prepared to feel slightly "lost" when you begin to relax. You are, however, perfectly safe – all that is happening is that you are undergoing a new (or old, but forgotten) set of sensations. Remember that everything that is happening as you relax is ultimately within your control. You can stop when you wish, restart when you wish, or even tense up again – if you wish.

It is crucial that you do find a way to rid yourself of tension, because only with the onset of relaxation can your body reverse

PROGRESSIVE MUSCULAR RELAXATION

This exercise helps you to recognize muscular tension as it builds up, allowing you to stop it before it becomes locked in. Results can come quickly – but only if you perform the exercise regularly!

1. Lie on a draught-free, carpeted floor, arms and legs out-stretched. Clench the fist of your dominant hand and hold tight for 10 seconds. Let go and enjoy the sense of release for 10–15 seconds. Repeat the action. Then, tense and release your other hand twice in the same way.

2. Curl the toes of the foot on the side of your dominant hand upward toward the sky. Hold for 10 seconds. Release and relax for 10–15 seconds. Repeat, then do the same to the other foot.

3. Perform the same sequence in at least 5 other sites, or pairs of sites, working up from your feet to your head. You could try, for example: pulling your kneecaps toward the hip to tense thigh muscles; squeezing your buttocks together; pulling your abdomen in strongly; holding a breath and at the same time drawing your shoulder blades together; tightening the face muscles around the eyes and mouth or frowning hard.

4. Practise daily for a week. Then begin tensing and relaxing groups of muscles together – all the muscles in the neck or chest, for example. After another week, abandon the tension element – simply focus on the different regions, note whether they are tense or not, and instruct tense areas to relax.

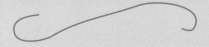

AUTOGENIC TRAINING

By following these steps for 10 minutes each day, you will learn to project certain sensations onto specific parts of your body, to relax them, to improve their circulation, or to relieve their inflammation.

1. Lie comfortably, with a cushion under your head, your knees bent and eyes closed. Focus on your dominant arm and silently say "my arm feels heavy". Sense the arm relaxed and heavy. For about a minute repeat the affirmation "my arm feels heavy". Your mind may wander periodically. Don't worry, this is normal – just return to your arm and its heaviness. Enjoy the sense of release – of letting go – that comes with this feeling.

2. Next, focus on your other arm and do exactly the same thing for about a minute.

3. Now focus your attention on your left leg, and then on your right leg, each time for about a minute. Repeat similar affirmations about the relaxed weight of your limbs all the while.

4. Return to your dominant arm and this time say to yourself "my arm is feeling warm". Apply this warming message to your 3 other limbs in the same order as before, focusing on each for about a minute. Feel the warmth, feel it spread, and enjoy the sensation it causes.

5. Focus on your forehead and affirm that it feels cool and refreshed. Hold this thought for a minute or so. Finally, stretch: clench your fists, bend your elbows and extend your arms.

the damaging hormonal processes that stress induces. Bringing about these positive biochemical changes will dramatically reduce your pain levels.

As a first step toward liberating ourselves from a state of tension we can use well-tried muscular relaxation exercise methods, the best known of which is called progressive muscular relaxation (see exercise, p.55). Other ways of releasing muscular tension, and so helping to calm the mind, include stretching methods (such as yoga and Muscle Energy Technique, see pp.87–91), biofeedback (see box, p.53) and autogenic training (see exercise, opposite), which combines elements of progressive muscular relaxation and meditation.

In time, if you become well practised in the progressive muscular relaxation and autogenic training exercises in this section, you will reach a point where you will be able to recognize tension building up, and will automatically, without even doing the exercises, be able to "switch it off". For example, with autogenic training you will be able to focus thoughts of heaviness into an area to dissipate tension. Autogenics can also be used to relieve pain caused by poor circulation (by focusing warm thoughts) or by inflammation (by "thinking the area cool"). This is a major step forward in pain control as well as in health enhancement.

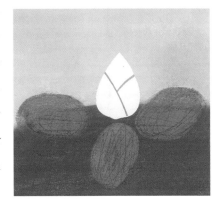

TAKING A BREATH

Although the two things may seem entirely unrelated, the way you breathe can have a fundamental bearing on your pain levels. Breathing in an incorrect manner can, over time, set in motion a chain of harmful mechanical, chemical and psychological reactions, which will make your symptoms worse, or may even have caused them in the first place. This section will show you how to identify whether you should change your breathing pattern, how to make any necessary alterations, and how to keep track of your progress.

In a normal, healthy breathing pattern, it is the movement of your diaphragm (situated below the ribcage) that makes your lungs inhale and exhale. However, in many people the role of the diaphragm has been taken over by the muscles in the upper chest. Breathing with the upper chest is normal when you are running (to clear build-up of acidic wastes), but not when you are performing everyday activities nor when you are resting.

A normal, uncontrolled diaphragmatic breathing cycle (in and out) takes about five seconds on average, making 12 breaths per minute, 720 per hour, 17,280 per day. If you use the upper chest to breathe, it is more than likely that you are a shallow breather, and so you will probably take considerably more than 20,000 breaths a day. The muscles that are stressed by such a strained and repetitive breathing pattern become tense and painful, and may develop trigger points (see pp.82–3). These muscles are the ones that lie between your shoulders and your neck and that attach to the neck, front and back, and to your ribs and shoulder blades. They are the very muscles that are often associated with chronic head and neck pain.

Breathing is not just about taking in the right amount of oxygen, but also about expelling the right amount of carbon dioxide. The carbon dioxide that you breathe out is derived from carbonic acid circulating in your blood. When you breathe rapidly, in an upper-chest pattern, you may get rid of too much carbon dioxide, and therefore too much carbonic acid, with the result that your blood becomes more alkaline. When this happens certain unwelcome changes take place, one of the most notable of which is that you become more sensitive to pain.

Another symptom of this condition is that your muscles become tenser and more prone to cramp, and feelings of pins-and-needles are common. In particular, when the smooth muscles around your blood vessels become tense, less blood (and, therefore, less oxygen) gets through to your muscles and to your brain. This causes tiredness and lack of stamina, as well as symptoms such as difficulty in concentrating and short-term memory lapses – often known collectively as "brain fog".

In addition, when your blood is excessively alkaline, your sympathetic nervous system becomes more readily aroused

BREATHE LOW

This exercise is designed to help you focus on 2 distinct ways of improving your breathing pattern. Steps 1 and 2 encourage the diaphragm to work properly. These steps are a good preparation for the core breathing exercise on p.63. Steps 3 and 4 will reduce the tendency of the muscles above the shoulders to contract during breathing. (This is a common sign of an upper-chest breathing pattern, particularly likely to affect people who work at a desk for long periods of the day.) You should do this exercise 2 to 3 times a day – you can practise the 2 halves separately, if you prefer.

1. Sit with one hand on the abdomen and the other hand on your chest, as in the hi-lo test (see opposite).

2. Breathe in through your nose and out through the mouth with pursed lips. As you do so, try to sense the movement of your abdomen – outward as you breathe in, and flattening again as you breathe out. Repeat this 5–10 times at your own pace.

3. Now, sit up straight with your hands on your lap, fingers interlocked, palms facing up.

4. As you inhale through your nose, push the pads of your fingers lightly but firmly against the backs of your hands to "lock" the shoulder muscles, preventing them from rising. Exhale through pursed lips and release the pressure in your fingers. Repeat this step at least 10 times.

(see pp.52–3), leading to a sense of apprehension and anxiety (and even panic attacks). In short, you will generally find that you are more easily upset than normal.

All of these symptoms are likely to be worsened when the upper-chest pattern of breathing coincides with a low-blood sugar episode, or the second phase of the menstrual cycle, which may explain some aspects of PMT (premenstrual tension).

With all this in mind, it is not difficult to see that increased pain, sensitivity and anxiety are the almost inevitable results of a breathing-pattern imbalance.

To find out what your breathing pattern is, try a simple exercise known as the "hi-lo" test. Stand in front of a mirror with one hand flat on your upper chest and the other flat on your stomach, just below your lowest ribs. Take a medium deep breath and see what your hands do. If the stomach hand moves first and there is not much movement at all of the upper hand, this suggests a diaphragmatic pattern, which is good news. If the upper hand moves first, and/or upward toward your chin, this suggests an upper-chest pattern of breathing.

The good news is that such a condition is not a disease, it is a pattern of use (like posture), and it can be fixed by substituting new patterns of use and behaviour. The exercises in this section are designed to achieve just that outcome – a new pattern of breathing to reduce anxiety and pain, and to deliver oxygen more efficiently to deprived muscles and brain tissues. By following these exercises for a month or two, you should notice an improvement in your breathing pattern. Use the hi-lo test again to see whether your inhalation is starting with movement of your diaphragm. When it is, the hand on your belly will move forward – not upward – at the start of the breath.

The following is another simple test you can use to help you monitor how well your body is adapting to higher levels of carbon dioxide, as your pattern steadily improves.

Breathe in normally and exhale, and time with a stopwatch (or a watch with a second hand) how long it is before you feel the need to breathe in again. If it takes less than 15 seconds, you are either an upper-chest breather or asthmatic. If it is between 15 and 25 seconds, you are average but still not quite at the ideal level, which is around 30 seconds. You should not try forcefully to hold your breath out, just hold until you have an urge to inhale (representing a message from the brain saying that levels of carbon dioxide are building up and that it's time to breathe again). Your body (and brain) may have become accustomed to low levels of carbon dioxide. As your breathing changes to a slower, diaphragmatic pattern, you will get used to higher levels. By carrying out this test on a daily basis and recording each day's result in your diary (see pp.32–5), you will build up a clear record of your progress and you will be able to gauge how positive changes in your breathing affect your experience of pain.

THE ETERNAL FLAME

Use this exercise both to counter feelings of anxiety and to reduce your pain levels. You should perform the full exercise twice a day – upon waking and just before bed. However, on a day when you are feeling particularly anxious, or when your pain is severe, you should also take a couple of minutes out of every hour to practise a shortened version.

1. Sit or lie down in a comfortable position. Imagine that there is a candle flame about 6 inches (15 cm) from your mouth. Exhale slowly and fully through pursed lips in such a way as not to "blow out" the imaginary candle. As you exhale, count silently to yourself to establish the length of the out-breath.

2. When you have exhaled fully, without causing any sense of strain to yourself, allow the subsequent inhalation to be full, free and uncontrolled. (The initial complete exhalation creates a "coiled spring", meaning that you do not have to tell yourself to breathe in – it happens automatically.) Count to yourself to establish how long your in-breath lasts.

3. Without pausing to hold the breath, exhale again – slowly, fully, through pursed lips, making sure to keep the flame alive.

4. Continue the inhalation and the exhalation for no fewer than 30 cycles. By the time you have completed 15 or so cycles any sense of anxiety which you previously felt should be much reduced. After several weeks of doing this exercise twice a day, you should achieve an inhalation phase of 2–3 seconds and an exhalation phase of 6–7 seconds – without feeling any strain.

THE POWER OF MEDITATION

Meditation involves focusing your mind on a single thing. In traditional meditation, practitioners concentrate on an idea or concept, for example, that God is love; or a word, such as "peace"; or an image – perhaps a candle flame. Another common focus for meditation is a mantra – a repeated sound or phrase (see opposite). Although many people associate meditation with mysticism and spirituality, one thing that it does not require is subscription to any particular belief system.

We can all train our minds to become completely absorbed in a task or a thought that is far removed from our pain. Studies show that simple meditations can turn a sufferer's attention away from the pain for up to 24 hours after the meditation session itself.

Meditation is one of the most effective means of producing a relaxation response to counteract the stresses associated with pain and anxiety. During meditation, brainwave patterns alter so that you remain awake and alert, but deeply relaxed, with your thoughts no longer dashing about from topic to topic. This often leads to a reduction in physical and mental tension, and an easing of stress-related symptoms such as high blood pressure, digestive problems and insomnia.

As with so many things, different forms of meditation suit different people – as well as the passive, reflective approaches outlined above, it is also possible to immerse yourself in a seemingly mundane activity to such an extent that it becomes a focus for meditation. You could meditate on painting a wall, doing the washing up, or even the simple act of breathing (see exercise,

REPEAT YOURSELF CALM

Meditating on a mantra – a repeated sound, word or statement – can be an effective way of stilling the mind, in order to reduce the feelings of anxiety that often breed tension and pain. Try practising the following exercise for 10 to 20 minutes daily.

1. Sit or lie in a comfortable position and let your eyes roll up toward your eyebrows.

2. Hold this mildly uncomfortable stare for about 30 seconds and then close your eyes and focus your mind onto a word or phrase. The mantra you choose may relate to your personal beliefs (for example, the Eastern "Om" or "Hare Krishna"; the Islamic "Allah"; the Jewish "Shalom"; or the Christian "Lord, have mercy"), or it could be a rhythmical word, such as "banana" or "coca-cola", that holds no particular significance for you. It is not the mantra itself but the repeating of it that makes it effective in quietening the chatter of the mind.

3. Say the mantra out loud – slowly, over and over, using it to gently override other thoughts that may enter your mind. Whatever mantra you choose will gradually become a droning sound in your mind as you repeat it. Imagine that this is the sound of a distant airplane, carrying away all of your unwanted thoughts, and leaving your mind quiet and still.

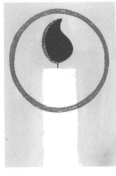

To feel the benefits of meditation, you should aim to meditate once a day – or twice if you are feeling particularly stressed. Each session should last between 10 and 20 minutes.

p.67). The only way to find out what suits you is to try various techniques and judge which make you feel most relaxed and clear in your mind.

Although they may differ in some respects, all meditation methods have certain basic requirements in common. Before embarking upon any meditation program, you should familiarize yourself with the progressive muscular relaxation, autogenic training and breathing exercises in the previous two sections, because during meditation your muscles need to be relaxed and your breathing regular and calm. You will need to find a quiet place in which you are unlikely to be distracted or interrupted. It is also important to choose a comfortable, balanced posture that you can hold for some time without feeling any strain – above all, ensure that you do not slouch. For example, try sitting up straight in a chair with your hands on your lap; or lying on a carpeted floor, perhaps with a book under your head to ease neck tension, your spine flat (put a small cushion under your knees if you have a hollow back).

The aim in meditation is to keep your mind focused on one object. However, you should not panic if you find that your attention wanders. Whenever you become aware that this has happened, you should simply refocus, gently. Visualize the uninvited thought as a pebble dropping into a pond. The ripples gradually get wider; as the surface becomes flat and calm again, you can refocus on your meditation object.

INSPIRED MEDITATION

The idea of this exercise is to breathe relaxation into tense, painful areas of your body. Follow these steps for 10 to 20 minutes each day.

1. Sit or lie comfortably and roll your eyes up toward your eyebrows. Hold this gaze for 30 seconds, then close your eyes and focus on your breathing: it should be relaxed and uncontrolled.

2. Count "one" on your first exhalation, "two" on the second, "three" on the third, and "four" on the fourth, then start again. Repeat this cycle throughout the meditation.

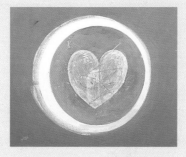

3. Become aware of the rising and falling of your abdomen. If your mind wanders, notice the distraction, then unhurriedly return to the counting and breathing.

4. After about 5 or 10 minutes, guide your breath to a painful area of your body. Imagine waves of cool air gently blowing away knots of tension in time with your counting and breathing. Then, steer your breath around the whole of your body, willing it to relax any other tight or uncomfortable areas.

THE MIND'S EYE

Visualization is a technique, allied to meditation, in which you create images or scenes in your mind and use them to positive effect – perhaps to bring about feelings of peace or to ease pain.

For example, you may wish to conjure up a "safe haven", either from your memory or your imagination. This might be a room, or a garden, or a riverside – anywhere that makes you feel content, peaceful and secure. The more vividly you evoke the scene, the more likely it is that you will achieve the desired effect. Therefore, you should try to draw on all your senses, building up layers of sights, sounds, smells and so on. For example, if you are imagining a garden you might first contemplate the neat stripes of a newly mown lawn, then the buzzing of the mower, the fresh smell of the cut grass, before walking out onto the lawn and feeling the sponginess of the grass under your feet.

Research suggests that visualization exercises work better if you prepare yourself, just before you begin, with a relaxation technique, such as autogenic training (see p.56), progressive muscular relaxation (see p.55) or breathing exercises (see pp.58–63).

Visualization can also be directed specifically toward health problems, as in the exercise opposite. You might wish to use surreal images, seeing a painfully inflamed joint as a bonfire which you extinguish in your mind with buckets of icy water; or you could envisage the angry red of the joint slowly fading to pink as you ease it with cooling breezes.

Once created, visualizations can be recorded onto audio cassette, so that you can return to them easily whenever you feel a need to retreat for a while from pain or anxiety.

WASHING AWAY PAIN

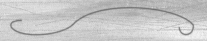

This exercise is a visualization in which you imagine raindrops washing away your pain. Read it slowly onto an audio cassette, embellishing it with your own ideas. When you are ready, play back the tape. Sit in a balanced posture (see p.66) – remember not to slouch. (If you lie down, don't fall asleep!)

1. Close your eyes and imagine that you are walking in your favourite park. Try to recall it in as much detail as possible. Use all your senses – conjure up smells and sounds as well as sights.

2. As you visualize yourself walking, imagine that your pain is rising to the surface of your body, transforming itself into pleasant, tingling sensations all over your skin. Your pain has migrated here. This is the first step in obtaining some relief.

3. It begins to rain – a few drops at first, becoming a shower. You don't mind the rain: it is warm, gentle and refreshing. After about a minute it subsides and then stops. Lift your arms and think about how they feel – the rain has "washed away" the prickling sensation on your skin. Be aware of your face – no more tingling there either. You have been cleansed of the worst of your pain: what remains is definitely diminished.

4. You feel jubilant and "light". Stay in your park for as long as you like. When you come out of your meditation, open your eyes and be happy that you still feel light and free. Smile. Carry this feeling of lightness with you for as long as you can.

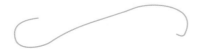

HEALING SOUNDS

Research suggests that listening to, or actually playing, music can induce various beneficial physiological changes, including slowing your breathing rate and heartbeat, reducing blood pressure and muscle tension, and influencing brainwave patterns in a way that improves your mood and eases stress. Sound waves can also be transmitted directly through the skin into problem areas by means of computerized devices. This can help to restore healthy resonance to an area that is out of rhythm with the rest of the body, thereby reducing pain.

If you are interested in the idea of music or sound therapy you could see a specialist, but equally there is much you can do at home. Simply select pieces of music that lift, hearten and relax you, and play them when you feel in need of encouragement, or as a background to your regular relaxation routine. It does not even have to be music – sounds such as wind-chimes, birdsong, waves breaking on the shore or the mellifluous voice of someone reading poetry or prose can all have beneficial effects.

Of course, we all have different tastes, so it would not be appropriate to suggest specific pieces of music. The important thing is that the music you choose strikes a chord with you. However, quite apart from personal preferences, it has been found that classical music works particularly well – even for people who claim not to like it.

BODY TUNING

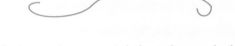

The following exercise uses music both to relax you deeply and to rebalance and reintegrate painful areas that may have fallen out of step with the rest of your body.

1. Sit or recline in a comfortable position, close your eyes and play a favourite piece of music that is at least 10 minutes long.

2. Sense your own body rhythms. Start with your breathing and your heartbeat before focusing on your inner energy system. Feel the energy flowing through your cells and organs.

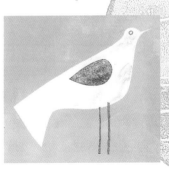

3. Now, focus on the music. Feel its rhythms merge with those of your body, so that you become part of the sound. Sense any discordant areas of pain and bring them into the same rhythm.

4. Feel at one with the music, absorbed by it, traveling with it, until it ends in silence and stillness. Let your body continue to vibrate gently with all parts now in harmony.

SLEEPING WITH PAIN

For sufferers of painful conditions, bedtime can bring with it apprehension and dread. Physical discomfort, and the anxiety engendered by it, often lead to insomnia. This section will show you how sleep works and what happens when it goes wrong, as well as outlining tried-and-tested strategies for improving the quality of your sleep – even if you suffer pain.

Insomnia? Don't lose any sleep over it!

Woody Allen (1935–)

Our brainwave patterns change during sleep as we pass through different stages, grouped into 90-minute cycles. The first phase within each cycle, called the *alpha* stage, involves light sleep, also known as REM (Rapid Eye Movement) sleep. This is when we dream. The next two phases are known as the *beta* and *gamma* stages, in which our sleep becomes steadily deeper. Finally, we enter the *delta* stage – the deepest and most restful period of sleep. During this phase, growth hormones, which are instrumental in the repair and healing of the body's tissues, are released by the pituitary gland.

Research shows that tissue-repair functions are most active between ten at night and ten the next morning. Therefore

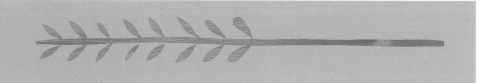

SLEEP-ENHANCEMENT STRATEGIES

There are many natural ways of improving your sleep pattern without taking prescribed medication. While they may increase overall sleep time, sleeping pills rarely address a deficiency in delta-stage sleep and they can be addictive. Try some of the following instead:

- *Ensure that your bedroom is neither too hot nor too cold – research suggests that a temperature of around 62°F (16°C) is generally conducive to sleep.*
- *Have a small, easily digested protein-rich snack, such as a yogurt, about an hour before bedtime, and avoid all forms of caffeine throughout the day. (However, avoid protein if you are having trouble digesting it.)*
- *Develop a bedtime routine to attune your body to expect sleep. This might include taking a shower or bath (using aromatherapy oils), reading, listening to music or performing breathing and relaxation exercises.*
- *For the hour before bedtime, reduce lighting levels and turn off the TV.*
- *If you wake during the night feeling alert, don't toss and turn – get up, go to another room, do a short relaxation routine, then go back to bed.*

(assuming we don't work the night shift), if sleep is disturbed, repair and recovery are likely to be delayed. When delta-stage sleep was artificially interrupted in research volunteers, a number of symptoms appeared within a few days, including tiredness, poor concentration and short-term memory problems – collectively described as "brain fog". When their sleep continued to be affected, the volunteers became withdrawn and felt pain in their muscles and joints. All of these symptoms disappeared when their delta-stage sleep was restored for just two nights.

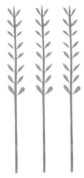

Nearly half of all sufferers of chronic muscular pain (such as fibromyalgia) experience disrupted delta-stage sleep. They are also likely to have low levels of serotonin, a compound involved in the initiation and maintenance of restorative sleep. When we are in good health, we make serotonin in our intestines from digested proteins. However, if protein digestion is poor, or the synthesis of serotonin is somehow disturbed, the consequences include disturbed sleep, a slowing down of the healing process and heightened pain perception.

In addition to the natural strategies suggested in the box on p.73, there are several herbal and mineral supplements that can assist in treating sleep problems. These should be taken only on the recommendation of a licensed healthcare provider. For example, a protein called 5-HTP (5-hydroxy-L-tryptophan) is said to encourage serotonin production, and is available in health-food stores. A combination of herbal products such as valerian, hops and passiflora can often ease sleep disturbances. Calcium and magnesium, taken together at night in a ratio of two parts calcium to one part magnesium, can alleviate muscular tension, and in so doing, remove another obstacle to healthy sleep.

Another treatment that has been shown to relax the nervous system, and therefore promote better sleep, is the "neutral bath" – a bath in which the water is at body temperature. Note that this treatment is not suitable for people suffering from serious heart disease, or skin conditions that react badly to water.

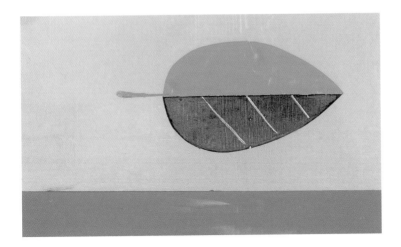

The only special equipment you will need for a neutral bath is a water thermometer. Before going to bed, run a bath as full as possible, with the water temperature as close as possible to 97°F (36.1°C) – and certainly no higher. When you get into the bath, the water should cover your shoulders. The effect of immersing yourself in water at this "neutral" temperature should be profoundly relaxing and sedating. Rest your head on a sponge or a towel. Keep an eye on the thermometer – the water temperature should not drop below 92°F (33.3°C). To adjust the temperature, top up the bath with warm water, but ensure that the temperature does not exceed the 97°F (36.1°C) limit.

The duration of the bath is up to you – anywhere from 30 minutes to two hours. The longer you spend in the bath, the more relaxing it is likely to be. Afterwards, pat yourself dry quickly and get straight into bed.

chapter four

BODYWORK AND REHABILITATION

Whether or not you require treatment for the cause of your pain, it is important that you are actively involved in your rehabilitation strategies. However, because carrying them out incorrectly can make your condition worse, you need to understand how your chosen technique or exercise discipline works, and apply guidelines accurately.

When you are recovering from pain and injury, or trying to maintain or improve physical function, you should perform exercises in a slow, fluid and measured way, avoiding stiff, jerky movements. The key features are control, concentration, rhythmic precision and repetition, with use of focused breathing to help coordinate movements. No matter what strategy you choose to follow – yoga, aerobic exercise, self-massage and so on – you will feel better far more quickly if you participate in your own recovery process in a focused and careful way.

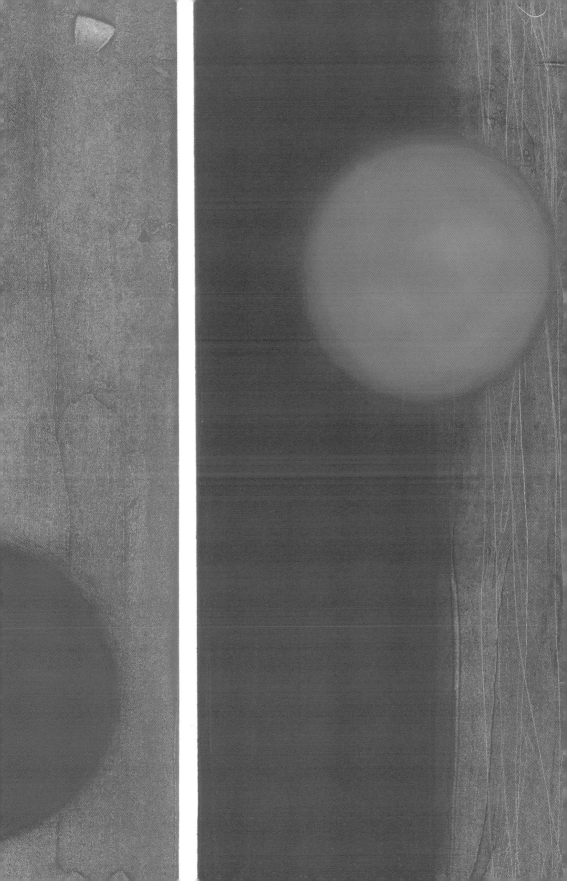

HEALING TOUCH

Rubbing a sore place to ease the pain is the simplest, most instinctive form of massage. This action and other massage strokes cause a variety of changes which are instrumental in reducing levels of pain and anxiety.

You can massage accessible parts of your own body – the next time you feel tense or have a headache, try making small circles on your forehead and temples with your index and middle fingers.

Not only does massage work on a mechanical level to relax tense muscles (and, therefore, ease discomfort), but it also provokes a series of beneficial neural and chemical reactions. For example, by stimulating nerve endings called *mechanoreceptors*, massage enables the brain to "shut the pain gate" (see box, p.18). In addition, massaging tissues causes them to release painkilling chemicals called endorphins, while the brain is encouraged to generate its own painkillers – enkephalins – as well as sleep-inducing serotonin. At the same time, massage has been shown to reduce levels of the stress hormone cortisol, thus easing anxiety and muffling pain perception. When correctly applied, massage also helps unblock the flow of blood and lymph around the body, so reducing the pressure in painful swellings and allowing fresh oxygen and nutrient-rich blood into irritated areas.

Research by Tiffany Fields, PhD, at the Touch Research Institute in Miami has shown that as few as two 30-minute massage sessions a week can significantly reduce the pain levels of sufferers of conditions as varied as fibromyalgia, arthritis, premenstrual syndrome, multiple sclerosis and migraine headaches.

Massage is suitable for almost everyone. However, you should not massage actively inflamed areas, open wounds or damaged skin. Another word of caution: if you are planning to receive massage from a professional therapist, you should first check that they are properly qualified.

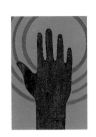

Although professional credentials are a useful indicator, an essential qualification for giving massage is a genuine desire to ease the pain of the recipient, which is why, for example, your partner or a close friend may be just the person.

A MASSAGE TO RELIEVE BACKACHE

The following example takes you step by step through a massage designed to relieve pain in the muscles of the middle back. If you have had no massage training, it is safest to use basic strokes such as *effleurage* and *petrissage* (these and the other main massage strokes are shown overleaf). To cut down on friction of hands on skin, apply a warm lotion or oil to the area you will be working on.

Kneel to the left of the person to be massaged – who should be lying face down on a bed in a warm, peaceful room. You should be perpendicular to him or her, with your knees pointing toward their flank. Using one hand in a slow, relaxed movement, reach across the person's back and push the muscles on the right-hand side of their middle back slightly down and away from you. The whole stroke should cover no more than 4–5 inches (10–12.5 cm). Ease your hand back to where it started while making a similar forward stroke with your other hand. Repeat the strokes to and fro so that your hands lightly wring the muscle. After a minute change sides and repeat.

common massage strokes

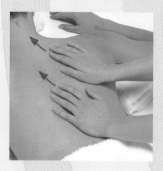

Effleurage is a light, gliding stroke, using the palm of the hand. One hand follows the other in a series of rhythmic, caressing actions. The stroke has a relaxing effect, and reduces fluid congestion by encouraging the flow of both blood and lymph.

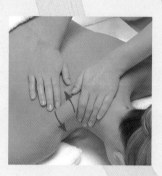

Petrissage involves lifting, pressing and rolling muscles in a movement akin to gently wringing out water from a damp towel. As one hand presses in one direction, there is a counter-pressure from the other hand which pulls in the other direction. The idea is to "milk" muscles of waste products and to stimulate circulation.

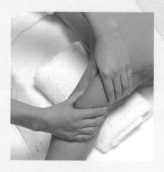

Kneading is a compressive stroke which squeezes tissues downward and then lifts them, in order to improve fluid exchange and to achieve muscle relaxation in the area. This can be compared with the hand actions involved in kneading dough when making bread.

Inhibition applies direct pressure to tender areas of tight muscles, often using a thumb. The pressure can be held for a minute or more – if this hurts, press for five seconds, ease off for a few seconds, and repeat for a minute, or until the muscle softens. The effect is to stretch tight muscles and to promote better circulation in the area.

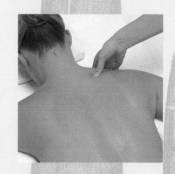

The **vibration and friction** treatment involves small, circular, vibratory movements, applied by the tips of the fingers or thumbs. This action has a relaxing effect and can ease chronic pain. Vibration can also be achieved with mechanical devices.

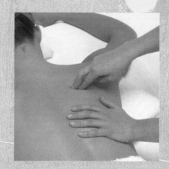

Feathering is a soothing method that is often used to conclude a massage session. It involves a series of light, overlapping strokes with the tips of the fingers, which brush like feathers slowly over the areas that have been treated.

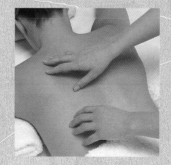

TRIGGER POINTS

Trigger points are localized, hyper-irritable areas of tension usually to be found in a muscle. They are created when a nerve ending (at the trigger point) becomes sensitized as a result of some form of emotional, mechanical or chemical stress – or a combination of these. Most people have such areas in the *upper trapezius* muscle, which lies between the neck and shoulder.

You can derive short-term relief of active trigger points by applying an ice pack to the painful area (see pp. 104–6).

Trigger points are so called because they are not only painful themselves when pressed, but – when they are active – they also provoke pain sensations some distance away from themselves, in "target" tissues. When a trigger point is not actively sending pain messages to a distant area it is said to be "latent".

Significantly, any stress affecting you as a whole – even something as seemingly unrelated as a climatic change or a sudden emotional event – may put strain on your muscles and, therefore, make trigger points more active.

The sorts of stress that are particularly likely to give rise to trigger points or aggravate existing ones include: mechanical wear and tear, owing to overuse of muscles, injury or poor posture; nutritional deficiencies (especially of vitamin C, vitamin

SELF-TREATMENT STRATEGIES

If you are suffering pain from an active trigger point, you may be able to deactivate it yourself for a short time, until you are able to deal with the underlying problem. First, you will need to find the trigger point. Carefully search the muscle that is aching – the trigger will feel swollen, stringy or nodular, and will be sensitive to finger pressure.

One of the most common locations for trigger points is the neck. To treat a point at the side or front of your neck, try to lift and squeeze it until you feel both the local pain and the target area symptoms. If the point is on the back of your neck or in the shoulder muscles, press into it with a finger or thumb. Hold for a minute. If this is too uncomfortable, press for five seconds, release for a second or two, then press again – repeat this cycle for a minute. Then, stretch the muscle (being sure to cause no pain) using MET (see pp.87–91).

B complex and iron); hormonal imbalances (low thyroid levels, or menopausal or premenstrual situations); climatic changes and cold draughts; infections involving bacteria, viruses or yeast; allergies; poor oxygenation of tissues; emotional tension; inactivity; and poor breathing habits.

The best way of deactivating trigger points is to get rid of the causes – for example, by improving your posture, breathing habits and diet or by reducing your anxiety levels. However, if you are already suffering pain from active trigger points, therapies that can help range from acupuncture to stretching and neuromuscular massage techniques (see box, above).

POSITIONAL RELEASE

Derived from osteopathy, Positional Release Technique (PRT; or "Strain-Counterstrain") can relieve pain by relaxing tight (short-ened) tissues and improving local circulation. Unlike massage and stretching, PRT is safe even on damaged or inflamed tissues.

Osteopathic medicine holds that many painful conditions result directly or indirectly from tissues (such as muscles, liga-ments and tendons) that have been strained, either quickly in a sudden incident, or gradually because of poor breathing, posture and so on. These strained tissues may stretch beyond their usual length – or they may become shorter than normal.

To ease discomfort in the chest owing to tight rib muscles, try applying PRT to tender points between the ribs in line with the nipple (for pain in the top four ribs), or between the ribs in line with the front of the armpit (for pain in the lower ribs).

What PRT illustrates is that if you gently ease tissues that have shortened to a position in which you make them even shorter, you can temporarily remove pain from the area. The exercise opposite shows how to use PRT on neck muscles, but you can adapt the steps to other areas. For example, if the pain-point is on the front of the body, bend forward to relieve it; the further it is to one side, the more you should ease toward that side. If the point is on the back of your body, ease slightly back-ward until the pain reduces a little, then turn away from the side where you feel the pain, and "fine-tune" to release the discom-fort. If the point is on a limb, try to shorten the relevant muscles (don't stretch them) by slowly moving the area to find the posi-tion in which the pain is most reduced.

FINDING A POSITION OF EASE

This experiment uses the sensitive muscles of your neck to show how PRT works. You can tailor it to any area, although you should not apply PRT to more than 5 pain-points in one day. If you follow these principles, your mobility should improve in a matter of minutes after the treatment, but it may take longer for pain to reduce. You may feel a little stiff or achy the next day, but this will soon pass.

1. Sitting in a chair, search for a place that is sensitive to pressure in the side of your neck, just behind your jaw, directly below your ear lobe. Press just hard enough to hurt a little, and grade this pain as a "10" (where "0" equals no pain at all).

2. While still pressing, bend your neck forward slowly. Keep deciding what the score is in the sensitive point.

3. As soon as the pain starts to ease, turn your head slowly toward the side where you feel the pain until the pain drops some more. By fine-tuning your head position, you should be able to get the score close to "0". Stay in this "position of ease" for about half a minute, then – very slowly – bring your head back up straight. The painful area should be less sensitive to pressure. If this really were a painful area, rather than an "experimental" one, the pain would ease over the next day or so.

1 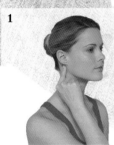 **2** 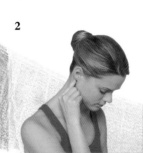 **3**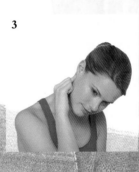

STRETCHING

Stretching is a natural means of restoring suppleness and free-dom of movement to areas of your body that have become restricted. It may also relieve the pain that so often comes with muscle tightness, especially if the condition causing the problem is chronic, or very acute (spasm or cramp, for example).

Stretching can be self-applied (active stretching), or it can be applied to you (passive stretching). Whenever possible, you should opt for the former – it is important that control should be vested in the hands of the person who can feel the effect of the stretch.

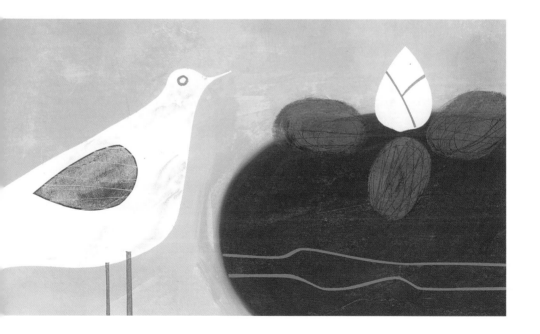

Because it is all too easy to overstretch, or to stretch too violently, we need to establish some basic principles. Above all, stretching should not hurt. If it does, you are performing the stretch wrongly, or too strongly. *Never* use force when stretching! If you force part of your body beyond its "barrier of resistance" (the point beyond which movement becomes uncomfortable), you risk exacerbating your condition. The day after you have performed stretching exercises, you may ache slightly, which is entirely normal, but your overall pain level should not have increased if you have stretched correctly. A final caveat is that you should not stretch inflamed tissues, or areas that have been injured within the previous three weeks or so, as this may interfere with ongoing healing and recovery processes.

There are many exercise systems that recognize the therapeutic value of stretching. Some use equipment, such as rubberized bands that offer resistance for you to work against. Other disciplines, such as Pilates, are founded on personalized instruction by a teacher. On the following pages we will look in detail at **yoga** and **Muscle Energy Technique** (MET) – two stretching methods that are safe, effective and easy to practise unaided.

The ancient Indian discipline **yoga** benefits the whole body in a variety of important ways, not all of which are immediately apparent. Most obviously, it helps to relax and lengthen tight or shortened muscles, and to mobilize stiff joints. Regular practice of yoga can also bring about improvements to your posture, thereby averting future musculoskeletal problems. With its emphasis on measured breathing, yoga also harnesses the stress- and pain-reducing effects of a healthy breathing pattern, leading to a calming of the nervous system. All of these positive factors work together to support the body's self-repair mechanisms and, therefore, to promote homeostasis (see pp.24–5).

The practice of yoga involves getting painlessly into specific postures (*asanas*). The postures look quite different, but they follow a similar pattern. In each case, the *asana* stretches a part, or parts, of your body to the barrier of resistance, but never beyond. If you find that you are using effort, and are feeling pain, you have gone past the barrier, and you should stop at once. Normally, you hold a yoga position, without effort, for some minutes, all the while breathing in a slow, relaxed manner. After a minute or two, you will usually have relaxed enough to move further in the direction of the stretch. You then hold this second position – again for a minute or two, by which time your muscles may have relaxed even further, enabling yet another increase in range. The exercise opposite shows you how to put these general principles into practice.

Like Positional Release Technique (see pp.84–5), **Muscle Energy Technique** derives from osteopathic medicine. MET involves identifying a muscle, or group of muscles, that is tense or shortened, and then using a very precise method for releasing any extra "tone" in the muscle to make stretching it easier.

THE TRIANGLE POSTURE

This yoga posture is an effective way of stretching the muscles on the sides of the body – perform it on both sides for a balanced effect.

1. First, stretch the right-hand side of your body. Stand with your feet about a yard apart, left foot turned fully left, and right foot slightly left. Extend your arms horizontally at the shoulder, palms facing down (a). Breathing out, bend to the left, so that your left hand can grasp your left leg as far down as is comfortable (b). As you bend, make sure you do not tilt forward or backward, and stretch your right arm toward the ceiling.

2. Now, turn your head as if to look at your right thumb. Your knees should not be bent at all, and your arms should reach as far as is comfortable. You should feel a stretching in those areas that are tight. Relax into this posture, breathing slowly.

3. After a minute, breathe out and, at the same time, ease your left hand further down your left leg, bending a little further to the left. Hold this position for another minute before slowly coming upright, and regaining your starting position.

4. Repeat steps 1–3 for the left-hand side of your body.

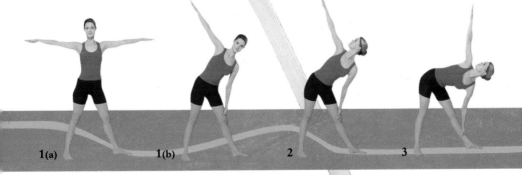

1(a)   1(b)   2   3

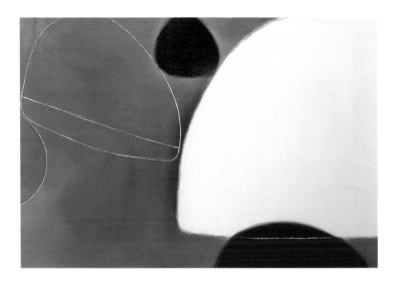

To achieve this result, the muscle needs to contract without being moved – this is known as an isometric contraction.

For example, if you sit at a desk or table and turn your head carefully to one side you will reach a point where it feels as though it will not turn any further without being forced (unless you are very supple indeed). Turn your head in this way, let's say to the right, and place your left elbow on the desk or table and your left hand flat against your left cheek. Now, using no more than a quarter of your strength, try to turn your head back to the centre, but prevent this movement with your left hand. The force of your turn and the force of the hand cancel each other out, bringing about an isometric contraction of the muscles that are trying to turn your head. This should not hurt – if it does, stop immediately. After about seven seconds release the effort and relax, breathe in and out and, as you exhale, see how much further to the right you can now turn your head without having to force it. (This muscle release is known as "post-isometric relaxation".) You have used MET principles on the shortened muscles that were limiting the movement of your head.

Interestingly, a contraction of precisely the opposite muscle will achieve a similar effect.

This time, still sitting at the desk or table, turn your head left until you feel a slight strain. Once again, place your left hand on your left cheek, and try to turn further left against the resistance of your hand, using a quarter (or less) of your neck-muscle strength. Again, hold for seven seconds or so, relax, and on breathing out see that you can now turn your head further to the left without effort. The muscle-release effect of using this method is known as "reciprocal inhibition".

Although these two variations achieve broadly the same effect, there are differences to bear in mind. Post-isometric relaxation has a stronger effect, but reciprocal inhibition is less likely to aggravate sensitive joints. As with any stretching method, you should not apply MET to inflamed or damaged areas.

You can follow the same procedure for any muscle that needs to be stretched: find the barrier of resistance; isometrically contract the muscles that are short; and after the contraction move more easily to a new barrier. MET is particularly recommended for relieving pain in muscles that house an active trigger point.

STAYING IN SHAPE

One of the most important aspects of recovery from pain is avoidance of what is known as "deconditioning". If you shun exercise in general, and specific movements in particular, because they hurt, or because you fear that they might hurt, you can easily fall into a habit of non-use. This can lead to a downward spiral, where your fear of pain leads to lack of activity, which results in deconditioning of your muscles, greater pain, and even greater difficulty in performing normal daily functions. This is a recipe for unhappiness and loss of self-confidence.

Regular exercise is invaluable in preventing or overcoming the effects of deconditioning, and ensuring that you maintain full body function. Exercise provides a mechanism to help you master any fear you may have of physical activity, and encourages you to take control of your pain. Through exercise you will also

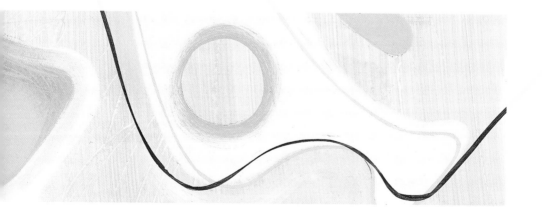

SET YOUR PULSE RACING

The beauty of the aerobic principle is that no matter how out of condition you are it can work for you. For a person who has just spent several weeks in bed, a slow walk around the room might raise the pulse rate to an aerobic-conditioning level. A more active person might need a fast jog around the park to achieve the same effect.

You can work out the pulse rate you should never exceed in your aerobic activity, and the pulse rate you should aim for, by feeding your age into the following simple formula:

- *To find your maximum pulse rate, deduct your age from the number 220. (Using a 40-year-old as an example: 220 – 40 = 180, so 180 is the pulse rate that this person should never exceed when exercising, in order not to strain his or her cardiovascular system.)*
- *To find your optimum exercising pulse rate, calculate ³/₄ of your maximum pulse rate. (In our example this is: 180 x 0.75 = 135, so 135 is the pulse rate that this person needs to achieve for 20 minutes three times a week to achieve aerobic fitness.)*

Walking is the best possible exercise. Habituate yourself to walk very far.

Thomas Jefferson (1743–1826)

cultivate and bolster your levels of motivation and self-discipline.

If you feel unsure about exercising, take heart: yes, pain is a warning to avoid stressing an area, but it seldom represents an absolute demand not to use the part at all, or the rest of your body as normally as possible. Clearly, there are exceptions, notably where you have been given medical advice to rest a part of your body (perhaps owing to a broken bone, a torn muscle or recent surgery). Sometimes you may even be advised to rest totally. But what is vital is that you do not make such decisions for yourself, avoiding activity to the extent of causing muscles to atrophy (waste) – rebuilding them can take many months of hard work! If you are in doubt, seek medical advice, but whatever you do keep using your body as normally as possible.

As well as helping you to develop a healthy, positive outlook, exercise can improve the functioning of your body systems. For example, thyroid hormone "works" better when you exercise aerobically – poor thyroid function has been linked to certain chronic pain conditions, such as fibromyalgia.

TAKE A BALANCED APPROACH

One reason often given for not exercising by people with impaired balance is fear of falling over. If you recognize yourself in this scenario, try improving your sense of balance with this simple routine.

Stand in a doorway with your arms folded (but ready to use the doorframe for support if needed). Looking straight ahead, lift one foot from the floor and see how long you can maintain this pose without touching the doorframe. If you can make it to 10 seconds, stand on the other leg and repeat the test. If you do not reach 10 seconds on each leg, practise several times a day until you can. Once you can balance on each leg for 10 seconds, do the same exercise with your eyes closed.

Your improved sense of balance will benefit you in everyday life – making walking and going up and down stairs easier. It will also make the prospect of aerobic activities much less daunting.

To reduce chronic pain symptoms through exercise, research has shown that you should follow a regular program, combining aerobic conditioning, flexibility work (stretching) and, if possible, strength-training activities. The aerobic aspect might include activities such as paced walking, climbing stairs, cycling, swimming or even non-impact aerobic classes. Other more creative possibilities include dancing, use of a mini-trampoline or skipping. The key is to tailor your program to your aerobic condition (see box, p.93) – with this in mind, you should check the suitability of any exercise regime with a qualified healthcare provider before embarking on it. It is probably best not to incorporate one-sided movements into your regular aerobic routine, so as not to create an imbalance. Above all, though, whatever forms of exercise you choose should be enjoyable, so that you see them as an integral part of your daily life, not as a tiresome intrusion.

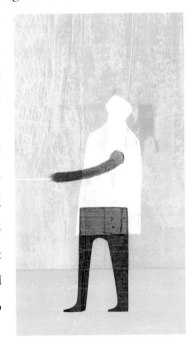

While stretching and flexibility routines are best followed daily, aerobic exercises are generally found to be most effective if performed three times a week, for approximately 30 to 45 minutes at a time. You should always carry out warm-up and warm-down stretching before and after aerobic activities, to avoid injury and to minimize stiffness.

chapter five

COMPLEMENTARY THERAPIES

Sometimes the rationale behind a given treatment is immediately apparent. If your shoulder were to ache, it would not take much to persuade you to have a massage. Similarly, a relaxation exercise would be a logical response to a stressful day. In this chapter, however, we will look at some less obvious therapies, such as acupuncture and aromatherapy, which can prove to be just as beneficial.

In evaluating some of the ideas presented here, try to get a feel for what attracts you, what makes sense to you, what you will feel comfortable with. You are not necessarily going to embrace all the methods outlined, despite some compelling evidence of their value. Only embark on those that you can accept intellectually – as we have seen in previous chapters, belief in a treatment is vital for its success.

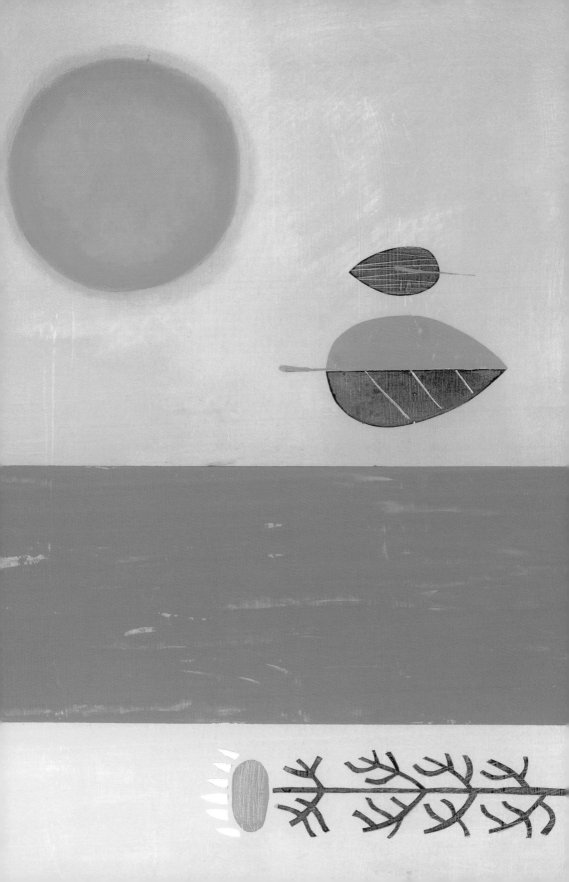

ENERGY AND HARMONY

Ancient Eastern concepts of vital energy form the basis of a wide range of therapies, such as acupuncture (see box, opposite), qigong and reiki. But how do they actually work?

Research into these treatments has demonstrated that they can benefit us in many ways. These include relieving anxiety, pain and chronic headaches, healing wounds, improving blood chemistry and correcting abnormalities in blood pressure.

Everything rests in prana, as spokes rest/ In the hub of the wheel…

The Prashna Upanishad

Significantly, studies have shown that such healing methods can also help enzymes, single-celled organisms, fungi, bacteria and plants to recover from exposure to x-rays or toxins. This proves that energy therapies exert a real physical influence, that they do not rely simply on the principle of "mind over matter".

A practitioner of, say, reiki can affect a patient's cells, blood and tissues without even touching the patient. This seemingly impossible phenomenon suggests that we need to revise our concept of the physical to take account of the effects of an invisible and intangible "energy".

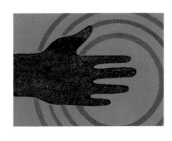

Eastern medicine has always incorporated the concepts of balance and imbalance of vital energy into its way of understanding health and disease. Known as *qi* in China, *ki* in Japan and *prana* in India, energy is seen as the feature that organizes all other body systems. It is the basis for therapies, such as acupuncture, that have been practised in the East for up to 5,000 years. Many of these therapies are now widely accepted in Western medicine because of their effectiveness, particularly in pain treatment, but with modern Western explanations replacing the traditional Eastern theories. We should not, however, simply discount the underlying beliefs of a system that has been in place since ancient times, especially now that research in quantum physics has provided insights that, in many ways, corroborate traditional Eastern energy concepts. The results of this research are already

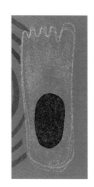

ACUPUNCTURE

The ancient Eastern therapy acupuncture is now widely practised in the West. It involves the insertion (usually quite painlessly!) of very fine, disposable, stainless-steel needles, into specific "points" on the body. Needles may stay inserted for a matter of seconds, or for 20 minutes or more, depending on what the acupuncturist is trying to achieve. Some traditional acupuncturists rotate the needles to produce a sense of heaviness in the area. A similar effect is achieved by modern acupuncturists, who pass mild electrical currents through the needles. Other methods of influencing painful tissues include heating the needles – this is known as moxibustion.

Western medicine believes that acupuncture operates by blocking pain messages to the brain (see p.18), in contrast to the traditional Eastern concept of acupuncture as an energy-rebalancing procedure. Regardless of the variations in belief and application, research has shown that this is one of the most effective methods for achieving pain relief – albeit temporarily if the causes are not also addressed.

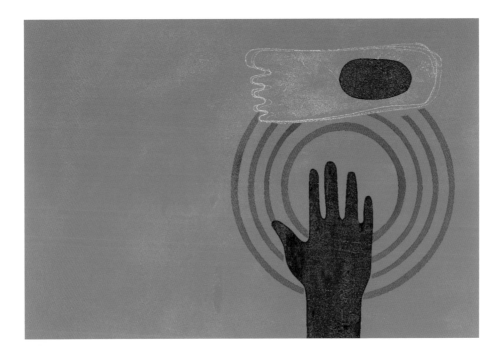

influencing Western medicine – as seen, for example, in the harnessing of biomagnetic fields to "jump-start" the healing of fractures, and in MRI (Magnetic Resonance Imaging) scans.

The old debate about whether there is such a thing as healing energy or life energy is being replaced by serious study of the interaction between biological energy fields, structures and functions, using instruments that are sensitive enough to detect the biomagnetic fields produced by the body's organs. Minute variations in light and heat emanating from the body can now be measured, and these can be related to different states of health and different stages of healing and tissue repair. Whether you prefer to think in terms of *qi* or of biomagnetism, do not over-look the huge number of therapies that are based on the con-cept of "energy" – they may be able to help you.

For example, practitioners of hands-on treatment methods, including osteopathy, physiotherapy, massage and craniosacral therapy, may unwittingly be using their own energy fields to help to balance those of their patients, thus encouraging the healing process. In contrast, martial-arts methods, such as aikido from Japan and qigong from China, train the individual to har-ness his or her own energy potentials, both for self-defence and overall well-being.

Energy modification is at the heart of systems such as reflex-ology, polarity therapy and reiki. This is also true of crystal ther-apy, and, to a large extent, treatments that use light and sound waves to promote health.

A rebalancing of energy fields may also be what is happening during the "laying on of hands" that forms a central part of spir-itual healing. This is widely practised by nurses in North America, where it is known as "therapeutic touch". The thera-pist's balanced energy rhythms are believed to merge with the unbalanced pulsations of the patient in a process known as "entrainment", with the result that the patient achieves a more harmonious energy pattern. The benefits of therapeutic touch have been shown to range from alleviating headache pain to reducing fever and inflammation.

Systems, such as reiki, that involve the channeling of healing influences from therapist to patient require that the therapist is in good health, and that he or she enters a state of centred, focused meditation as they embark on the healing or balancing procedure.

LIGHT AND COLOUR

Seasonal Affective Disorder (SAD), which leads to the "mid-winter blues", is the condition that most clearly tells us just how important it is to have regular, direct exposure to natural daylight. Research in Florida has also demonstrated that muscle strength is significantly reduced when daylight, or full-spectrum artificial light, is deficient. In addition, there is evidence that lack of light can lead to increased fatigue, irritability and attention lapses, all of which can be reversed by correcting light exposure. The implications are obvious for anyone who is house- or bed-bound because of illness or pain.

A variety of hormonal imbalances may also arise when we are deprived of light. This is because the pituitary gland, which influences all hormonal functions, has an absolute need for what is termed "full-spectrum light". This is only available to the pituitary if light enters the eye without having been filtered through glass. Full-spectrum light differs from the light emitted by most incandescent and fluorescent sources, which almost always lack the blue and ultraviolet end of the spectrum. As mentioned, a major factor in reducing your pituitary gland's access to light is spending too much time behind glass – at home, in office buildings, in the car, or wearing wraparound spectacles (or contact lenses). Even being outdoors on a sunny day may not help if you are wearing sunglasses,

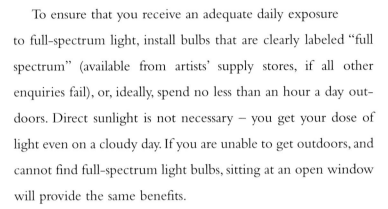

especially if they are tinted pink or orange, because of the wavelengths that are screened out. Blue-tinted glasses are less of a problem.

To ensure that you receive an adequate daily exposure to full-spectrum light, install bulbs that are clearly labeled "full spectrum" (available from artists' supply stores, if all other enquiries fail), or, ideally, spend no less than an hour a day outdoors. Direct sunlight is not necessary – you get your dose of light even on a cloudy day. If you are unable to get outdoors, and cannot find full-spectrum light bulbs, sitting at an open window will provide the same benefits.

During a meditation exercise, try visualizing a particular colour streaming into you, or seeing yourself bathed in that colour. Imagine blue if you feel a need to be calmer, red or yellow if you want to energize yourself.

COLOUR THERAPY

In Ayurvedic (Indian) medicine, different energy centres in the body, known as *chakras*, are said to respond to different parts of the spectrum. For example, the throat *chakra*, which is believed to have particular influence on the thyroid gland, and to be in need of balancing in cases of insomnia or overactivity, would be treated with blue light. This might call for wearing blue clothing, using blue-coloured light bulbs or drinking water that has been exposed to blue light.

There is no strong evidence for coloured-light therapy affecting physical symptoms directly. However, mood and emotion, which can certainly influence our sense of well-being, do seem to be helped by exposure to different-coloured lights. Canadian and American research has shown that exposure to yellow and red lights produces definite stimulating effects, while blue and black lights are calming.

HYDROTHERAPY

Hydrotherapy has been used for centuries for pain relief, and is still a popular rehabilitation treatment in spas and hospitals. Water has remarkable properties, not just in its liquid state, but also as ice and steam. It has an amazing capacity for transferring heat, whether this involves bringing warmth to a body part or cooling it. When we move in water, our weight is partially supported by the liquid, so that exercises that might otherwise be impossible can be performed painlessly.

One of the most versatile and easily administered hydrotherapeutic treatments is the ice pack. Because of the large amount of heat it absorbs as it turns from solid back to liquid, ice can dramatically reduce inflammation and the pain it causes. Use ice packs for all sprains and recent injuries, joint swellings (unless you find that the ice aggravates the pain), bites, headaches, toothaches and hemorrhoids. Avoid using ice on the abdomen if you have an acute bladder infection, or over the chest if you suffer from asthma, and stop using it immediately if you find that the cold aggravates your condition.

To construct an ice pack, first place a layer of crushed ice – at least 1 inch (2.5 cm) thick – onto a towel. Fold the towel over the ice and pin the fabric together with safety pins. Lay a cloth made of wool or flannel over the area to be treated and put the ice pack on top, covering it with plastic to hold the water in.

CONSTITUTIONAL HYDROTHERAPY

Constitutional Hydrotherapy (CH) has a non-specific "balancing" effect on the body as a whole. When it is used daily or twice-daily for several weeks, CH can induce relaxation, reduce chronic pain and enhance immune function. To apply CH you will need: 1 double sheet folded in half, or 2 single sheets; 2 blankets (wool, if possible); 3 large bath towels; 1 hand towel (half the size of the bath towels); and hot and cold water. You will also need help to apply CH, and the instructions in this exercise are addressed to your helper.

1. The patient should lie undressed, face up between the sheets and under a blanket. Fold back the top sheet and the blanket, then place 2 folded bath towels that have been soaked in hot water (and partially wrung out) directly onto the patient's trunk, covering him or her from shoulders to hips. ("Hot" means too hot to leave your hand in the water for more than 5 seconds.) Cover the patient again with the sheet and blanket and leave them like this for 5 minutes.

2. Fold back the top sheet and the blanket, then place a hot-soaked hand towel on top of the "old" bath towels and flip all the towels over so that the hand towel is next to the skin. Remove the old towels. Place a cold-soaked towel onto the new hot towel and flip again so that the cold is on the skin. Remove the hot towel. Re-cover the patient with the sheet and the blanket, and leave him or her until the cold towel warms up. If the patient complains of feeling cold, massage their back, feet or hands.

3. Remove the previously cold, now warm, towel and turn the patient over. Repeat steps 1 and 2 on the patient's back.

(You should also ensure that surrounding clothing and bedding are protected from melting ice.) Bandage the whole package in place and leave it for about 20 minutes. Repeat the treatment after an hour if it proves to be helpful.

Another therapy, the sitz bath (derived from the German for "to sit"), is used to stimulate circulation. There are various ways of taking a sitz bath, depending on the equipment that you have available, but in any event you will need two containers. The ideal containers would be old-fashioned hip baths, but, failing that, you could use plastic bowls that are large enough for you to sit in with room to spare. Half fill one of the baths or bowls with hot (but not boiling) water, and half fill the other with water that is as cold as possible. Sit in the hot water – it should come up to your navel – and put your feet in the cold water. After three minutes, switch bowls as quickly as you can, so that you are now sitting in the cold water with your feet in the hot water, and stay like this for a further minute. Repeat these steps once from the beginning, then dry yourself and go to bed, either for an afternoon nap or for your night's sleep.

One caution is necessary regarding the use of heat. Although comforting, heat of any sort tends to cause tissue congestion. As with the sitz bath described above, where hot water is used it should always be followed by cold or cool applications, which decongest and restore normal circulation to the tissues. This is crucial if you are to get the best results from hydrotherapy.

COLD ("WARMING") COMPRESS

This is an ideal self-treatment for any of the following: painful joints; mastitis; a sore throat (compress on the throat from ear to ear and held by a strap over the top of the head); backache (ideally the compress should cover the abdomen and the back); and a sore, tight chest caused by bronchitis. As the compress slowly warms, the effect is deeply relaxing and pain diminishes. If you find the compress soothing, use it up to 4 times daily for at least an hour at a time. Ideally leave it on overnight.

You will need the following equipment: a piece of cotton large enough to cover the area to be treated (double thickness for people with good circulation and vitality, single for those with only moderate circulation and vitality); a single thickness of woollen or flannel material large enough to cover the cotton (a towel will do but is not as effective); a piece of plastic of the same size as the wool or flannel; safety pins; and cold water.

1. Wring out the piece of cotton in cold water so that it is damp but not dripping. Place it over the painful area and immediately cover it with the woollen or flannel material and the plastic. Bandage it snugly in place, so that it is airtight, but not so tight as to impede circulation.

2. The cold material should rapidly warm and feel comfortable. If the compress is still cold after 20 minutes it may be too wet or too loose – remove it, give the area a brisk rub with a towel, then replace the compress, making any necessary adjustments (wringing it out more or bandaging it more tightly).

3. Wash the material before reuse, as it will absorb body wastes.

NATURE'S BOUNTY

Aspirin, originally derived from willow bark, is an example of the contribution plants have made to modern medical science. However, natural does not always mean safe – arsenic is as natural a herb as you can find. All the same, those herbal medicines that have been well researched, and their safety proven, produce fewer adverse physical reactions than pharmaceutical drugs. The following are examples of herbs commonly used for pain relief.

Aloe vera gel has an antiseptic effect when applied to wounds, burns, stings, bites, ulcers and abscesses. The gel can be taken directly from the cut leaves of the plant for external use, or purchased in a preparation to be taken internally to soothe most digestive disturbances.

Cayenne pepper and **red chilli pepper** extracts, rubbed onto the skin, can ease pains such as those left over after shingles, or those linked to most chronic (but not acute) joint problems.

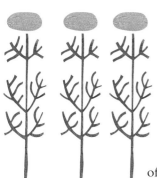

Chamomile is known for its anti-inflammatory and antispasmodic properties. It can be taken as an infusion, or applied on a compress, or it can be used to bathe the eyes.

Clove oil is applied directly onto painful dental sites where its anesthetic properties produce rapid relief.

Comfrey (once known as "knitbone") has a long history of use in treating burns, bruises, sprains and fractures.

DECOCTIONS, TINCTURES AND INFUSIONS

Herbs are commonly taken in the form of decoctions, tinctures and infusions. These preparations are all simple to create.

To make a **decoction** of berries, roots or bark, place the herbs in a saucepan, cover them with cold water, and bring to the boil. Simmer until the liquid reduces by about a third, before straining into a container for storage in a cool place.

A **tincture** is made by soaking the herb in a spirit (typically vodka) for two weeks to extract the active ingredients. The herbs are then sieved through a muslin-lined wine press, and the resulting liquid stored in dark-glass bottles.

An **infusion** is made in much the same way as tea. Cover the herbs with boiling water and let them infuse for about 10 minutes. Strain into a cup and drink. You may need to add a small amount of honey to make the infusion palatable.

Cramp bark has strong anti-spasmodic properties, making it ideal for all forms of spasmodic cramp, especially if you have also suffered an emotional upset. The herb can be taken as a decoction or a tincture (see box, above).

Ginger relieves digestive pain. Take either as an infusion or in the form of a capsule, available from health stores.

Ginkgo biloba can be taken in capsule form for conditions such as intermittent claudication and other problems involving poor circulation.

Marigold (calendula) ointment soothes cuts and grazes.

HEALING SCENTS

Essential oils should be stored in dark-glass containers, in a cool place that cannot be reached by children. The oils should be discarded when they reach their expiry date.

Aromatherapy involves the therapeutic use of essential oils that are extracted from plants such as rose, lemon and lavender. Each has specific properties, such as the ability to encourage relaxation, reduce anxiety or alleviate fatigue. Oils can be administered in a variety of ways: they can be added (sparingly) to a bath, massaged into the skin, inhaled directly or diffused in a room.

The role that essential oils can play in pain relief is well documented. Arnica has been shown to ease the pain caused by labour, chemotherapy and surgery. Lemon and lavender oils can help us cope with stress of any sort, including pain.

AROMATHERAPY FOR ANXIETY

The following combinations of essential oils have been used successfully in massages to combat stress and anxiety symptoms. In each case the mixture should be diluted in 1 fl oz (25 ml) of base oil.

- *For feelings of tension and anxiety linked to muscular pain and discomfort mix together 10 drops of clary sage, 15 drops of lavender and 5 drops of Roman chamomile.*
- *For apprehension associated with fear and foreboding mix 15 drops of bergamot, 5 drops of lavender and 10 drops of geranium.*
- *For anxiety associated with chronic fatigue, poor concentration and insomnia blend 10 drops of neroli with 10 drops of rose otto and 10 drops of bergamot.*

Indeed, lavender is one of the safest, most commonly used and most versatile oils for pain relief. To soothe burns and insect bites, it can be applied undiluted to the skin and covered with a dressing. For aches and pains, try adding a few drops to a cold "warming" compress (see p.107). Other ways of using lavender oil include: tipping a few drops onto a handkerchief or ball of cotton wool and inhaling from it; pouring 10 drops into your bath; and diffusing it into your room using a steam inhaler or 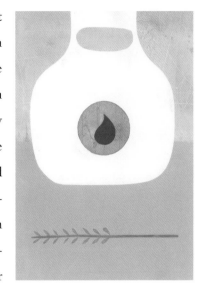 a diffuser. In addition to its direct pain-relieving properties, lavender also increases alpha waves in the brain, which promote relaxation and deeper sleep.

Aromatherapy is safe, requires no costly equipment and is easy to practise in the home. However, there are some guidelines that you should bear in mind, in addition to the manufacturer's instructions. When applied directly to the skin, all oils (except for lavender) must be diluted in a neutral base oil, such as almond or sunflower. It is important to test for allergic reactions before trying a new oil. Put a drop on the skin on the inside of your elbow and wait 24 hours to see whether you develop a rash. You should never take oils internally or apply them to the eyes, and pregnant women should avoid aromatherapy altogether, unless prescribed it by a licensed healthcare provider.

chapter six

EATING WELL

The expression "you are what you eat" is close to the truth, for the raw materials we take in through food and drink provide the building blocks of everything that we are made of, and they fuel every process that takes place in the body. Inflammation and tissue healing can be helped by good nutrition, or slowed down by a deficient diet. Biochemical disturbances, resulting from food allergies and intolerances, can cause pain or aggravate existing pain.

The information in this chapter is for guidance only. Dietary changes are most safely accomplished when you obtain advice specifically related to your condition from a qualified and licensed practitioner. However, one step that you are urged to take is to use your pain diary (see pp.32–5) to test the effects of any changes to your diet. Relying on memory alone is not a good idea. The diary, with data recorded daily (ideally at the same time each day), gives you a definitive record from which to work.

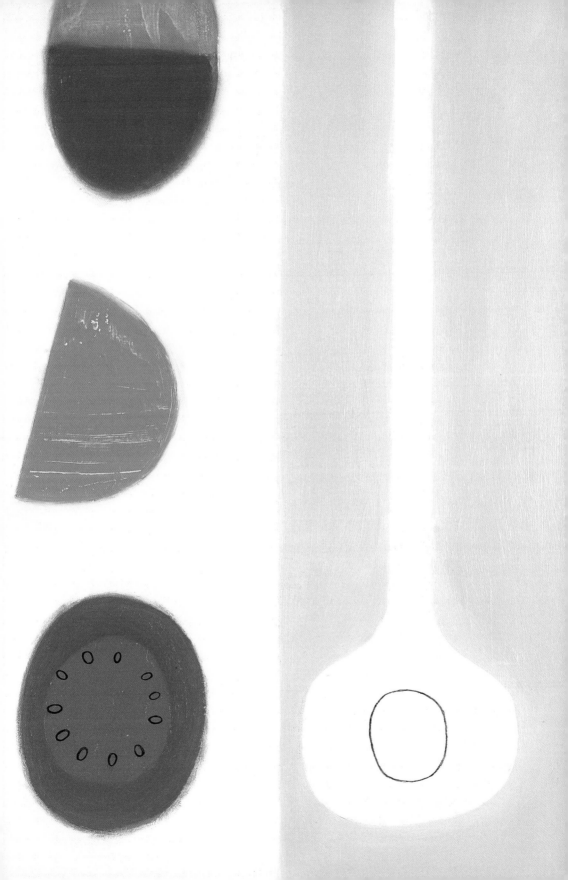

INFLAMMATION AND DIET

What we eat can have a marked impact on the inflammation process (see p.29). One of the most important ways of using your diet to control inflammation requires a two-pronged approach. This calls for increasing your intake of fish oils (because they contain eicosapentenoic acid, or EPA, which calms inflammation) and reducing consumption of meat and dairy fats (because they contain arachidonic acid, which fuels inflammation).

Eating fish from a cold-water source (such as the North Atlantic, or the waters off Alaska) two to three times weekly should provide you with a good amount of EPA, especially if the fish is of an "oil-rich" variety (for example, salmon, herring, mackerel or sardine). If you do not eat fish, you can obtain EPA capsules from any pharmacy or health-food store – ask a qualified healthcare adviser what dose is appropriate for you.

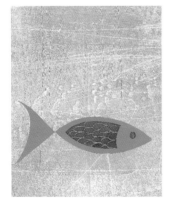

To reduce your intake of arachidonic acid, you do not necessarily have to avoid eating meat altogether. Certain types of meat, such as game birds and poultry – above all, turkey – are relatively low in fat, especially if you don't eat the skin. However, duck and goose are fatty meats – try to avoid them.

Of course, the only fail-safe way of preventing your intake of animal fats from affecting your health is to avoid eating any animal products whatsoever.

DAIRY-FREE ALTERNATIVES

Giving up dairy products in order to cut down on inflammation-inducing animal fats does not mean you have to give up milk, ice cream and cheese. There are many delicious alternatives to try.

Instead of animal milk *try plant milks, such as rice milk, soy milk, nut milk (almond or cashew) or oat milk (but not if you are on a grain-free diet)*

Instead of ice cream *try fresh-fruit sorbet, frozen or fresh-fruit smoothies, juice popsicles, fruit ice cubes, frozen rice desserts (made from rice milk), frozen tofu desserts, fat-free yogurt*

Instead of cheese *try tofu, fat-free cheese*

Research has shown that a vegan diet (no animal or fish products at all) can have beneficial effects on inflammatory conditions such as rheumatoid arthritis, leading to reduced pain, swelling and stiffness. (You can also derive benefit from a low-fat vegetarian diet, incorporating 2–3 ounces (60–90 g) of low-fat cheese or yogurt daily, and eggs from time to time.)

You should think hard before adopting a vegan diet, and – as with any any major dietary change – it is important to make your decision in consultation with your physician and a nutritional expert. With a limited range of dietary choices, vegans run the risk of developing certain nutritional deficiencies. However, if you follow a balanced, well-planned pattern of eating, including

– if necessary – supplementation of those elements
that are likely to be missing (see p.125), there is no reason
why you cannot make a vegan diet work for you.

If you are vegan (or are considering becoming so to help
manage your pain) you should take special care to include protein in your diet. By combining different vegetable sources, it is
perfectly possible for vegans to obtain appropriate amounts of
protein. For example, eating any two of the following three types
of food in the same meal provides the necessary materials to
generate protein: grains (such as wheat, barley, oats, rye or rice);
pulses from the bean family (such as soy, lentil or chickpea); and
seeds (such as sunflower, pumpkin or sesame). Try a meal of lentil
soup with bread, or of tofu (which is made from soy) and rice.

Another system that has been shown to help dampen down
inflammation is the macrobiotic diet. This is a Japanese approach
to eating which borrows the Chinese concepts of *yin* and *yang*.
The idea is to balance your intake of calming *yin* foods, such as
green vegetables and fruits, with stimulating *yang* foods, such as
grains, root vegetables and fish. The macrobiotic diet may be
founded on traditional Eastern concepts, but it fits in very well
with the anti-inflammatory strategy of moving away from high
meat consumption toward eating more fish and vegetables.

You can also alleviate the pain caused by inflammation
by harnessing the effects of catalysts known as enzymes. Your
stomach depends on these enzymes, some of which are

AN ANTI-INFLAMMATORY DIET

These examples of seasonal meal plans show how you can exclude animal products from your diet and still consume a balanced range of nutrients.

SUMMER

Breakfast
Cereal (granola), fruit and nuts with 1 cup plant milk (e.g. rice or soy milk)

Mid-morning snack
Mixed-vegetable drink

Lunch
Cool soup: cucumber or gazpacho, and vegetable salad with olive oil OR tofu pâté, bean spread or hummus, 1 cup potato, and wholegrain bread

Mid-afternoon snack
Banana or grapes

Evening meal
Variety of steamed vegetables, and wholegrain pasta with sauce OR cold-potato, grain or bean salad and raw-vegetable salad with olive oil

Late-evening snack
Fruit sorbet OR frozen soy yogurt

WINTER

Breakfast
1 cup oatmeal with 1 cup plant milk

Mid-morning snack
Warm tomato juice with rye crispbread and tahini

Lunch
Warm soup: miso, bean or vegetable, and fresh salad dressed with olive oil and lemon juice OR baked beans and tofu with wholegrain bread

Mid-afternoon snack
Herb tea with dried fruit

Evening meal
Lentil soup, steamed vegetables and baked potato OR baked tofu, 1 cup mixed grains and raw-vegetable salad with an olive oil and lemon dressing

Late-evening snack
Rice cake with pureed-fruit spread

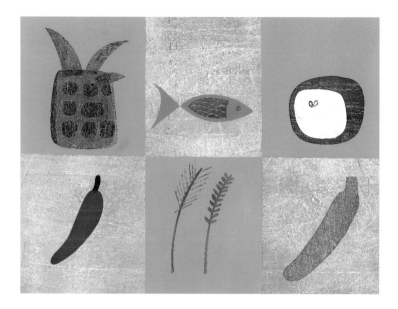

produced by your pancreas, to digest the food that you eat. For example, there is an enzyme called lipase that helps the digestion of fats, and another called lactase that helps you process dairy foods. Proteolytic enzymes stimulate protein digestion. Some foods, such as pineapple and papaya, contain high levels of these enzymes, and can be used to tenderize protein-rich foods – for example, by wrapping meat in papaya leaves before cooking.

Proteolytic enzymes also have a gentle anti-inflammatory effect – particularly bromelain (derived from the pineapple stem) and papain (from the papaya plant). You can obtain these two enzymes in capsule form (available from health-food stores). To help reduce inflammation, try taking 2–3 grams of bromelain or papain in separate doses through the day, away from meal times.

OTHER DIETS AND PAIN

The range of health diets available can be bewildering – some popular examples that have been designed to counter specific types of pain, or pain in general, are briefly summarized below.

The **anti-candida diet** is a strict low-sugar, low-yeast regime. It aims to control overgrowth in the body of naturally occurring yeasts such as *candida albicans*. Yeast overgrowth may trigger a variety of allergic reactions and also pain in muscles, joints and the digestive tract (as well as the genital organs if thrush is a feature). Although the diet seems to be effective, many people follow it needlessly, because they misdiagnose themselves as suffering from yeast overgrowth. Expert advice is called for.

A great step toward independence is a good-humoured stomach.

Seneca
(*c.* 4BCE–65CE)

If you are suffering pain as a result of toxicity of any sort, a **detox diet** may help cleanse your system and support liver function. This may involve fasting or consuming only raw food or juices for a period. However, seek expert advice – a detox diet is unsuitable for many groups of people, such as those taking prescription medication or those who are severely underweight.

The **Hay diet** – said to increase energy levels and reduce pain – is named after its creator, Dr William Hay. A key part of the method involves not eating proteins and carbohydrates in the same meal. There has been no scientific validation of Hay's ideas – any benefit may actually derive from the increased attention that followers of the diet give to what they eat.

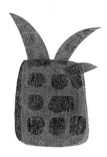

THE EXCLUSION ZONE

Adverse reactions to particular foods and drinks are responsible for a great deal of pain and discomfort. Headaches, constipation or diarrhea, vomiting, muscle and joint pain, tiredness, skin irritations, palpitations and agitation are just some of the symptoms that these reactions may provoke. Even when they are not the root cause of pain, allergies and intolerances may aggravate existing painful conditions. It can be difficult to identify foods that

THE NIGHTSHADE FAMILY

Research has confirmed that foods derived from the nightshade family can increase pain levels in some people. The members of this food group include: tomatoes, potatoes (but not sweet potatoes), aubergines (eggplant) and peppers (but not black pepper). Note that tobacco is also a nightshade plant.

If you are in pain and wish to test the possibility that nightshade foods are affecting you, leave them out of your diet for two weeks. During this period note your pain scores and symptoms in your diary each day. If you are sensitive to these foods, you should feel the benefit four or five days after excluding them. If after two weeks you feel that your pain has reduced, start to eat the foods again regularly for a week and note whether your pain increases. If so, this confirms that you should exclude nightshade foods from your diet for several months before retesting your reaction to them. If you feel no benefit from the two-week exclusion then continue to eat these excellent, nutritious foods as normal.

may be adding to your pain. In this section we describe the most reliable method of pinpointing any culprits – namely, excluding foods and drinks from your diet, then recording in your diary any subsequent changes to your pain levels.

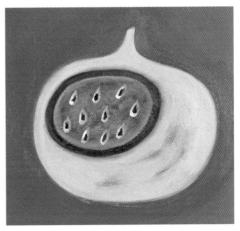

Adverse food reactions seem to be split into two categories – true food allergy (hypersensitivity) and the far less understood phenomenon of food intolerance. Research suggests that food intolerance may result from food toxicity, or it may be that the sufferer is deficient in the enzyme, or enzymes, required to digest a particular food.

Food reaching the digestive system is usually broken down by enzymes into molecules. Some of these molecules, containing nutrients, are transferred across the lining of the intestines into the bloodstream. Other, larger molecules, containing waste products, are eliminated from the body. However, sometimes the gut wall becomes irritated, which allows the larger, waste molecules into the bloodstream. Known as leaky-gut syndrome, this influx of undesirable molecules into the blood can lead to a variety of painful symptoms involving joints and muscles. Drugs and toxins (such as antibiotics, steroids and alcohol), advancing age, pesticides or additives in food, chronic constipation,

Chemicals in instant coffee (but not in regular-brewed coffee) can inhibit the function of endorphins – natural painkillers produced by the body. Try not drinking instant coffee for a few weeks, noting pain levels in your diary.

emotional stress, and major trauma, such as burns, can all contribute to the transfer of waste products into your bloodstream.

Research has identified the foods and drinks that are most likely to aggravate the symptoms of people suffering from chronic muscular pain. These are: wheat and dairy products, sugar, caffeine, artificial sweeteners, alcohol and chocolate.

If you suffer from chronic pain symptoms, you may benefit from conducting a food-exclusion experiment. To be able to draw firm conclusions from such an exercise, you should

THE EXCLUSION DIET PART ONE: PLANNING

1. List any foods or drinks that you know disagree with you, or that produce allergic reactions (skin blotches, palpitations, tiredness, agitation or other symptoms).
2. List any foods or drinks that you consume at least once a day.
3. List any foods or drinks that you would really miss if they were no longer available.
4. List any foods or drinks for which you sometimes have a definite craving.
5. Which foods or drinks do you use for snacks?
6. Which, if any, foods or drinks have you begun to consume more often/more of recently?
7. From the following list, highlight in one colour any items that you consume every day, and in another colour any that you consume three or more times a week: bread (and other wheat products); milk; potatoes; tomatoes; fish; cane sugar or its products; breakfast food; sausages or preserved meat; cheese; coffee; rice; pork; peanuts; corn or its products; margarine; beetroot or beet sugar; tea; yogurt; soy products; beef; chicken; alcohol; cake; biscuits (cookies); citrus fruits; eggs; chocolate; lamb; artificial sweetener; soft drinks; pasta.

approach it methodically. Try using the exclusion diet below, or the oligoantigenic diet on p.124, to structure your investigation.

Bear in mind that when you stop eating a food to which you may be sensitive, and which has been a regular part of your diet, you may experience withdrawal symptoms at first, including flu-like symptoms, muscle and joint ache, and anxiety and restlessness. Any side-effects will usually pass after a few days, and can be a strong indication that you may well be allergic to, or intolerant of, whatever it is that you have just cut out of your diet.

THE EXCLUSION DIET PART TWO: ACTION

1. Exclude from your diet the item you have listed most often in part one. If there is a tie for first place, it doesn't matter which you choose to exclude first – toss a coin if you like.

2. If after a week your symptoms (muscle or joint ache or pain, fatigue, and so on) have improved, you should maintain the exclusion for two or three weeks more, before reintroducing the excluded food or drink to see whether the symptoms return. If they do, and you feel as you did before the exclusion period, you will have confirmed that your body is better off, for the time being at least, without the food you have identified.

3. Repeat the exclusion process for the next-most frequently listed item on your questionnaire. Work down your list, always choosing the next-most frequently mentioned item.

4. Remove from your diet any items that tested "positive" in your exclusion experiment. Wait at least six months before retesting the problem foods or drinks. By then you may have become desensitized to them and be able to tolerate them again.

THE OLIGOANTIGENIC DIET

Another way to identify foods to which you are sensitive is to try a modi-fied oligoantigenic exclusion diet. Exclude at the same time for three to four weeks all the foods and drinks listed below as "forbidden". If you feel less pain after this period, reintroduce items that you had previously eaten, one at a time, leaving at least four days between each reintroduction. If, when you reintroduce a particular food, your pain symptoms recur, eliminate that food from your diet for at least six months. Allow five days for your body to clear all traces of the offending food before continuing the gradual reintroduction of the remaining excluded items.

Fish: white fish, oily fish allowed; smoked fish forbidden.
Vegetables, pulses: none is forbidden, but people with bowel problems should avoid beans, lentils, Brussels sprouts and cabbage.
Fruits: all are forbidden, except banana, passion fruit, peeled pear, pomegranate, paw-paw and mango.
Cereals: rice, sago, millet, buckwheat and quinoa are allowed; wheat, oats, rye, barley and corn are forbidden.
Oils: sunflower, safflower, linseed and olive are allowed; corn, soy, "vegetable" and nut (especially peanut) are forbidden.
Dairy: all dairy is forbidden – including cow's milk and all its products and all goat-, sheep- and soy-milk products.
Drinks: herbal teas are allowed; tea, coffee, fruit squashes, citrus drinks, apple juice, alcohol, tap water and carbonated drinks are forbidden.
Miscellaneous: sea salt is allowed; all yeast products, chocolate, preservatives, all food additives, herbs, spices, honey, eggs, most margarines, and sugar of any sort are forbidden.

SUPPLEMENTS

We have already seen that boosting your intake of EPA (found in fish oil) and certain enzymes can ease pain, because of their natural anti-inflammatory properties. There is also strong evidence in favour of supplementing other nutrients to help ease pain – ranging from calcium and magnesium to various B-vitamins, and essential fatty acids found in evening primrose oil.

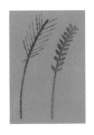

However, you will only benefit from taking a supplement if you are deficient in the nutrient in question in the first place. As a result, it is not always advisable to self-prescribe nutrient supplements. For a start, supplements can be expensive, and buying those you do not need unnecessarily costly. Secondly, certain vitamins and minerals, such as selenium and vitamin B_6, can cause toxic reactions if you exceed the recommended dose. To get the most out of supplements, you should consult a licensed nutritional expert, such as a dietitian, nutrition counsellor or naturopath. By seeking expert advice you will avoid falling into the trap of unnecessary, and potentially unbalanced, supplementation.

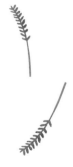

Having said that, there is certainly no harm in taking a well-formulated multivitamin or multimineral supplement to ensure that at least the basic requirements of the body are being met. And calcium and magnesium will aid muscle and bone health, particularly if taken pre- and post-menopausally by women to protect against osteoporosis in later years.

chapter seven

TYPES OF PAIN

There are pains that can be described as a "nice hurt" (as in deep massage, for example, when the therapist's hands are satisfyingly touching the source of discomfort), and some that are a background nuisance, or that are so familiar and non-threatening that they can almost be ignored. And then there are the pains that are awful, that dominate all thinking, and that prevent normal functioning. And there are pains that lie somewhere between these extremes.

Benjamin Franklin said that the only two certainties in life were death and taxes, but he could have added pain to his uncomfortable list, because none of us escapes it. This chapter presents examples of types of pain, from the everyday to the severe, and offers specific advice on how to ease them. The hope is that with increased understanding of the choices available, pain can be handled as effectively as possible, leaving time to concentrate on paying taxes!

READING THE SIGNS

One way of looking at pain is as the body's means of communicating distress. Pain speaks in many different ways – it may shriek at you, or nag, or grumble. By heeding the tone and nuances of this language, you can gain important insights into the nature of the condition affecting you, and plan your recovery accordingly.

Some pains are clearly local, and have little bearing on your general state of health. Strains, sprains, burns, bruises, joint injuries and localized osteoarthritic changes, resulting from overuse or injury, can all be treated for what they are – local conditions. Acute local conditions will usually recover in a matter of days or weeks, as long as they are not aggravated during the recovery phases of the natural healing process. Local arthritic problems – involving, say, a wrist or a knee – need to be evaluated to see how you can modify everyday patterns of use to reduce stress on the joint. You should also consider whether these problems can be helped by strategies such as hydrotherapy, acupuncture, exercise, direct manual treatment, medication or changes to your diet.

Other pains may derive from conditions that affect the body as a whole. In these cases, you will invariably need to adopt a broad-based approach, taking into account nutritional, emotional, hormonal, circulatory and other bodywide influences. Examples of generalized pain-producing problems include rheumatoid arthritis and fibromyalgia, which require

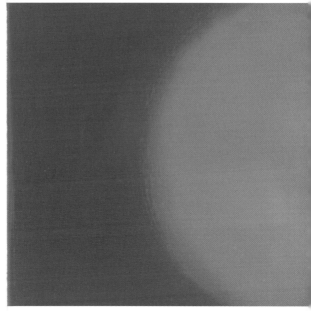

treatment of the whole person – mind as well as body. (They may also call for local treatment to ease particular symptoms.)

Other forms of pain combine both local and general elements, for example sciatic pain down the leg derived from a back condition; or trigger-point referral patterns, where the pain is felt in one place, but comes from a trigger in a distant muscle; or a headache originating from neck strain. Working with a healthcare professional, you need to trace these pains to their source, so that the causes can be addressed – dealing with them locally is not the solution.

As well as working out whether a pain is local, general or referred, you should assess whether it is acute or chronic.

Treatment strategies will vary depending on the answers you give to the questions in the box opposite. If your condition is acute, you should not apply any treatment that might increase inflammation or other acute symptoms, or that might interfere with the healing of tissues. Chronic problems, however, require a different approach. For example, in order to ease pain caused by joints or muscles that have tightened over time, you might try regular focused stretching, exercises and strengthening methods.

A word here about inflammation. This is a key aspect of the recovery and healing processes, and, as such, you should respect it. However, if inflammation is causing pain, you should aim to reduce it through natural strategies, such as hydrotherapy or dietary changes, rather than by resorting to medication (see p.28).

There are many strategies that can offer a measure of relief from all kinds of painful conditions. Examples include relaxation methods, better nutrition and aerobic activity, all of

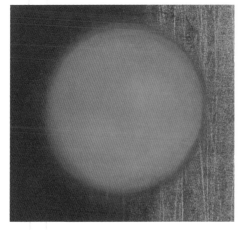

which have universal effects on the body by reducing stress levels, improving circulation and making the body's defence-and-repair systems run more efficiently. And there are also the numerous specific and local methods, discussed elsewhere in this book, that can help as first aid, or provide short-term relief.

MAKING SENSE OF YOUR PAIN

It is important to analyze your pain in a methodical way, either to prepare yourself for a consultation with a healthcare practitioner or to devise your own self-help strategies. Considering the following questions will help you to organize your thoughts.

- *What has caused my pain?*
- *Is it local/part of a general condition/a combination of the two?*
- *Has it been referred to the area that hurts by another part of my body?*
- *Is it acute/chronic/an acute flare-up of an old (chronic) problem?*
- *If the pain is acute, is the painful area inflamed?*
- *What eases the pain? What aggravates it?*
- *What can I do to aid the healing process? What should I avoid doing?*
- *How can I best engage my inner resources to deal with my pain, and to overcome the restrictions it imposes on me?*

The built-in ability of the body to recover from illness and impaired function is the greatest health-guarantor we have. This is the "physician within", working tirelessly toward recovery, which we can assist by removing obstacles to health, and which we need to harness when we begin to feel despair.

Quite apart from specific therapies, all of which can be helpful, the three key features examined in chapters one and two are essential for the tackling of any type of pain – we need to understand the pain process, achieve some control over it, and exert the powerful command of the mind over the body.

COMMON PAINS

Thankfully, most people's experience of pain is restricted to minor bumps, bruises, stings, cuts and burns. Listed here are some of the most common causes of "minor" pain, together with first-aid measures that may prove to be helpful.

To treat **bruises**, dissolve one or two arnica triple-strength homeopathic pillules (available from many pharmacies) under your tongue every 30 minutes until discomfort starts to ease.

When tackling a **burn or scald**, first remove the source of the burn and any clothing or jewelry in the area of the injury. If the burn was caused electrically, seek emergency assistance. If the area involved is less than an inch (2.5 cm) across, treat it yourself. If larger, get expert help. Place the burn under cold running water immediately and keep it there for no less than 10 minutes, longer if possible, or until medical help arrives. Never use butter, oil or grease on a fresh burn and do not break any blister. Cover with a light gauze bandage until you receive expert advice. Use a diluted lavender-oil dressing once healing is underway.

To relieve **muscle cramp**, either stretch the muscle immediately or find the centre of the cramp and apply strong thumb pressure until it eases. Check your nutritional balance, particularly of sodium and magnesium, with a qualified practitioner.

To get to the root cause of a **mouth ulcer**, you will probably need to seek medical advice. However, first aid may be

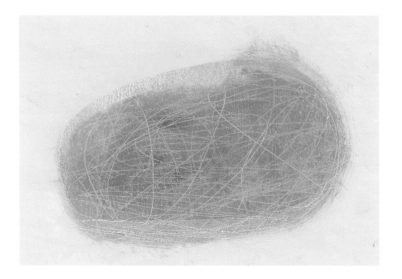

helpful: place a moistened tea bag over the ulcer for as long as possible; or suck an ice cube, trying to keep it over the ulcer site.

Steam inhalation is a useful first aid for easing painful **sinus inflammation**. Pour boiling water into a bowl and add a drop of pine or eucalyptus oil. Place your face over the bowl, with a towel draped over your head, for 10 to 15 minutes. Repeat this treatment several times a day.

Insect stings are most commonly inflicted by bees and wasps. If stung by a bee, remove the sting using tweezers (with wasp stings there is nothing to remove). Place the area under cold running water for at least 10 minutes and then apply vinegar or lemon juice, or a bicarbonate of soda paste, to neutralize the venom. If there is any sign of an allergic reaction – say, difficulty breathing or swallowing – seek urgent medical attention.

A PAIN-BY-PAIN DIRECTORY

On the following pages we take a tour of the body's major trouble spots, in each case looking at how pain most commonly arises there and suggesting appropriate therapies and strategies from earlier chapters.

headaches

Headaches are common, and usually not life-threatening. However, it is wise to get medical advice if a headache is out of the ordinary (for example, accompanied by visual disturbances, high temperature, very stiff neck, throbbing, or if the pain comes on after a sudden head movement or blow to the head).

The pads of a TENS unit (see box, p.18), applied either to the sides of the head or to each side of the neck near the base of the skull, can ease tension headaches, but not migraines or cluster headaches.

There are three main types of headache. A **tension headache** is characterized by aching (seldom throbbing) and a feeling of tightness in the temples (or the top, or back, of the head), as well as discomfort in the neck and/or shoulders.

The classic **migraine** is usually one-sided, with severe pain (throbbing, pounding or piercing) lasting for many hours or days. Migraines may be heralded by an aura of flashing lights, or by nausea or extreme sensitivity to light. The cause of migraines remains unclear – they may be triggered by weather changes, or bright or flickering lights, or stressful episodes. If attacks coincide with menstruation, hormonal irregularities may be the cause.

Like migraines, **cluster headaches** are usually one-sided, but, unlike most migraines, they start without warning. Typically lasting about an hour, they involve severe pain in the eye, temple, face and neck, and sometimes the teeth and shoulders. Cluster headaches are more common in men and are often accompanied by sweating and a running nose or eyes, suggesting a food intolerance or allergy background (see pp.120–24).

Some treatments are appropriate for all three types of headache. These include relaxation and visualization methods, especially autogenic training and biofeedback (they only work for migraines if you apply them at the first sign of the headache). Certain aromatherapy oils – particularly lavender and

Over-the-counter painkillers and prescribed migraine drugs can help to ease headaches. However, most carry the risk of side-effects, such as nausea and drowsiness. Migraine medication also seems to increase the frequency of attacks.

HOW TO AVERT A TENSION HEADACHE

If applied before the headache is well established, this method can ward off tension headaches, but not migraines or cluster headaches.

- *Place 2 gallons (9 litres) of hot water (not scalding) into a bowl large enough to accommodate both feet. Stir 1 to 2 teaspoons of mustard powder into the bowl and immerse your feet, up to the ankles.*
- *Wrap a large bag of frozen peas in a towel and place this behind your neck. (If you sit on an upright chair against a wall, you can lean back onto the towel containing the peas.)*
- *Spend at least 10 minutes in this position and then lie down and rest.*

chamomile – can assist the relaxation process, as can soothing herbal teas, such as chamomile, rosemary, lavender and ginger. Acupressure (see p.138) and acupuncture can also be effective, although for migraines you will usually need to follow a full course of acupuncture.

There are certain therapies that work particularly well for tension headaches. For example, many tension headaches derive from trigger-point activity, and so may benefit from manual treatment of the muscles housing the triggers (see pp.82–5). Hydrotherapy can often help – particularly the alternating of hot and cold applications to the back of the neck, or a cold compress to the forehead or back of the neck combined with a hot foot bath (see box, p.135). At the simplest level, you should keep warm and rest, eat only light foods and avoid alcohol.

Rest is also an important way of combating migraines, although, rather than keeping warm, you should lie down in a cool room. Other strategies include massage and manipulation – especially of the upper-neck area – using osteopathic, chiropractic or craniosacral methods. Studies have shown that these techniques can prevent migraines (in some cases permanently),

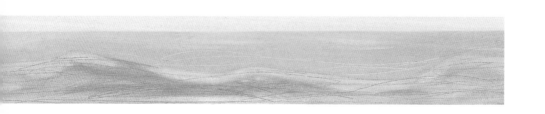

and may also help abort attacks once they have started. Pressing on pressure or trigger points on the temple or base of the neck may be effective, especially if the pressure initially increases or reproduces your symptoms.

Herbal feverfew tablets (or eating one feverfew leaf daily, if you grow this rather bitter herb) have been shown to reduce the frequency and intensity of migraines for some people, but are of no help once a migraine has started. Advocates of another complementary therapy, homeopathy, claim good results with migraines – but you should seek expert advice, rather than going it alone.

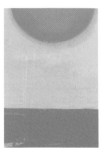

Although distinct from migraines, cluster headaches respond to all the treatments and self-help methods suggested for migraines.

Certain foods appear to provoke migraines, so a record in your pain diary of everything you have eaten in the 12 hours leading up to an attack may help in the detective work. Key suspects include: alcohol; tyramine-rich foods (such as mature cheese, chocolate and some nuts); nitrite-rich foods (including most cured or preserved meats); foods rich in monosodium glutamate (MSG); and artificial sweeteners. Following an oligoantigenic diet may help you find the culprits (see p.124). Low-blood sugar episodes (hypoglycaemia) seem to provoke migraines in some people, suggesting that you should not skip meals, and that you should follow a balanced diet that excludes high-sugar items. Deficiencies in specific minerals and vitamins may also be a factor. However, you should consult a qualified nutritionist rather than prescribing yourself supplements.

jaw, face and tooth pain

Pain in, or deriving from, the jaw (temporomandibular joint, or TMJ) can be severe. TMJ syndrome may involve difficulty in opening the mouth fully and in chewing, as well as noisy cracking and grating in the joint. There may also be active trigger points in the jaw muscles, which can be treated manually using neuromuscular massage, pain-killing injections or acupuncture.

Try these first aids for toothache: wash your mouth frequently with half a teaspoon of salt (or five drops of myrrh tincture) dissolved in a glass of warm water; or apply clove oil or brandy to the painful area using a cotton-tipped applicator. TENS and acupuncture can also help in the short term.

The causes of TMJ pain include dental imbalances (malocclusion), which can be corrected by certain dental practitioners, especially those who offer craniosacral therapy. Postural habits that stress the neck and head – for example, sitting with round shoulders and head forward – may also be to blame. If this is the case, you should consult a chiropractor, specialist osteopath, physiotherapist or an expert in postural retraining, such as an Alexander Technique teacher. Habitual tooth grinding (bruxism), often linked with anxiety, is another potential factor – it can be countered by wearing a plastic guard, especially at night. Relaxation, autogenic training and visualization will help ease the psychological stress that can be the root cause of TMJ problems.

Pressing the acupuncture points in the webbing between the thumb and index finger of each hand, closer to the finger than the thumb, can relieve toothache, headache and TMJ pain. Press firmly with your other thumb for up to a minute at a time. (Do not press areas of inflammation, broken skin or varicosed veins.)

A TRIATHLON FOR YOUR JAW

This 3-stage routine for alleviating TMJ pain is easy to carry out yourself – try it 3 times a day. Although the effects vary from person to person, you could expect to notice a reduction in your jaw pain after about a week.

1. Sit with one elbow on a table, and your clenched fist supporting your jaw. Gently try to open your mouth against the resistance of your fist, which should slow the opening but not stop it altogether. Open and close your mouth 5 times, and then open and close it 5 more times without the hand resistance. Make sure the lower teeth stay behind the upper teeth on closing.

2. Relax, then slowly open your mouth as far as you can without pain to stretch the muscles controlling the jaw. Hold for 5–10 seconds. Repeat this stretch once.

3. Sitting up straight, place the tip of your tongue as far back on the top of your mouth as you can. While the tongue is in this position, slowly and gently open and close your mouth a few times as widely as you can without causing pain. This activates particular muscles (the retrusive group) and helps to reduce tension in them.

neck and shoulder pain

Many kinds of neck pain, including whiplash injuries, may involve activated trigger points. Try using Positional Release Technique (see pp.84–5) to treat these trigger points.

Unless you have suffered a specific injury (see below), pain in the neck and shoulders usually comes from a habitual posture that puts stress on the muscles in this area. The most common culprit is a round-shouldered, head-forward posture, which not only strains the muscles supporting and moving the neck, but also crowds the upper chest, causing breathing imbalances. As muscles gradually become more tense they also develop trigger points, which can refer pain into distant tissues (see pp.82–3).

Treatment should aim to stretch the tightened muscles, deactivate trigger points, tone up weakened muscles and improve posture (see opposite). Physiotherapists, chiropractors, specialist osteopaths and neuromuscular massage therapists can all help.

Another common cause of neck and shoulder pain is "whiplash". Often these injuries heal within a few months. In other cases damage occurs to delicate nerve structures, disks and joints, leading to long-term pain and restricted mobility. In a few cases, small muscles at the base of the skull are so severely affected that they atrophy, which can give rise to fibromyalgia (see p.152). If you have a whiplash injury that is still uncomfortable, you are strongly advised to consult an expert. Self-help steps that may aid your recovery include: acupuncture and TENS; anti-inflammatory nutritional and hydrotherapy measures; and relaxation and visualization exercises.

REBALANCE YOUR POSTURE

Many of us spend long periods of our working day at a desk, hunched over paperwork or a computer keyboard. These, among other activities, can lead to an unbalanced, round-shouldered posture that pushes your head forward. The following exercise should help to ease the muscles in the neck and shoulders that are stressed as a result of such a posture. Do it hourly during time you spend working at a desk.

1. Perch on the edge of a chair or stool, with your feet flat on the floor, slightly wider apart than your hips, toes pointing slightly outward.

2. Tucking your chin in slightly, allow your arms to hang down with your palms facing forward.

3. Breathe in normally. As you breathe out turn your arms anti-clockwise so that your thumbs face backward and stretch out your fingers. At the same time, lift your breast bone slightly forward and up, and very slightly arch the lower back. Relax, and repeat 5 times.

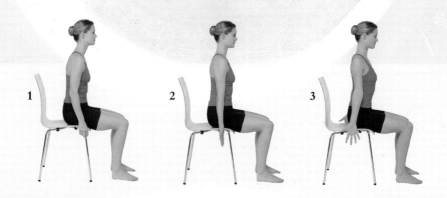

arm and hand pain

The arms and hands are particularly susceptible to repetitive strain injuries, which include tenosynovitis ("tennis elbow") and carpal tunnel syndrome (affecting the hand and wrist). If you work at a desk, you can take 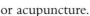 steps to minimize your chances of developing such conditions: avoid typing for more than four hours a day; stretch for three minutes every half hour; pay attention to your posture, the height of your desk and the position of equipment such as your computer; undertake general, regular exercise; and monitor your stress levels.

If you do develop an "overuse" problem, it can be treated with rest (and sometimes splinting of the wrist), physiotherapy or even surgery (for example, to release trapped nerves). If the area is inflamed, reduce swelling through diet and hydrotherapy (especially an ice pack). Any trigger points giving rise to the pain should be deactivated, for example using neuromuscular massage

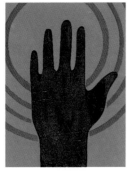

or acupuncture.

If the condition is severe, cortisone injections may be an appropriate option. However, repeated application can weaken tissues. Before resorting to cortisone, you should try conservative methods, such as ergonomic and postural re-education, TENS, acupuncture and bodywork – under expert supervision.

"TENNIS ELBOW" RELIEF

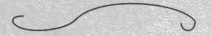

This exercise uses MET (see pp. 88–91) to relieve the pain in the inner elbow associated with "tennis elbow". (This condition can be caused by any activity that leads to overuse of the elbow joint – not just playing tennis.) If you do the exercise no more than once a day, you should feel benefit after about a week.

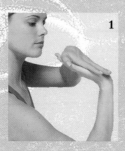
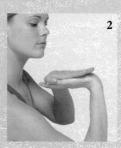

1. Sitting with your painful elbow on a table, forearm upright, palm facing forward, gently bend your wrist back with your other hand, so that your fingers point toward your head. Bend only as far as you can without it hurting. With your wrist in this bent position, use your other hand to resist an attempt to bring the wrist back to its neutral position. Maintain this light isometric contraction of the flexor muscles in your forearm for 7–10 seconds.

2. Relax, and then press lightly on the palm of the hand being treated to bend it back further than was possible in step 1. Stretch the flexor muscles in this way for at least 20 seconds.

3. Repeat steps 1 and 2 at least once more.

backache

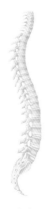

No pain provokes more visits to the doctor than backache, although – even without treatment – it usually gets better within a few weeks. However, if pain persists, you must seek professional advice, as the list of potential causes is so varied – including disk problems; trapped nerves; irritated, blocked or inflamed joints; muscular irritation or spasm; or trigger-point activity. Occasionally, persistent back pain can be caused by other internal problems, such as kidney disease or a gall-bladder condition.

Advice for backache will depend on its cause. However, there are some general principles. Above all, do not do anything that aggravates the pain. It is important to work out the difference between "hurt" and "harm". Hurting is OK if it is doing no harm. For example, gentle back stretches (see exercise, opposite) may hurt, but as long as they do not aggravate your existing back pain, they are unlikely to be doing harm – and may well help.

Avoid complete rest unless this is advised by an expert, or unless pain is extremely acute. If you do not use your muscles, they can rapidly lose mass and strength, which will slow down your recovery. Similarly, avoid using a back support for more than a few hours at a time, unless advised otherwise by an expert. Long-term recovery from chronic back pain almost always demands the strengthening of spinal and abdominal stabilizing muscles – this requires expert advice and instruction

Looked at in profile, the spine is curved in an "s" shape. When you stand up straight (when your earlobe is directly over your instep), the natural curves of your spine are properly supported by your back muscles.

STRETCHING YOUR BACK

Stretching may ease your back pain if the problem appears to be muscular. This exercise is a simple example of the kind of stretch that is often effective. However, if you find that it aggravates the pain, do not proceed any further. If, on the other hand, the exercise does seem to help ease your back pain, perform it 2 to 3 times each day. To prepare for the exercise, apply an ice pack to the painful area for 5 minutes, or use an ice spray for 5–10 seconds.

1. Lie on your back on the floor, knees bent, with your feet flat on the floor and a hand on each knee. Breathe in, then as you exhale draw your stomach down toward your spine. At the same time, use your hands to pull your knees toward your shoulders (not your chest) until you feel a stretch, but not pain, in your back. Hold this position while breathing normally, with your lower abdomen pulled in toward your spine, for a further 4 to 5 breathing cycles (in and out).

2. Then, as you exhale try to draw your knees a little further toward your shoulders. Hold this for 3 minutes and then relax with your knees bent, and your feet flat on the floor.

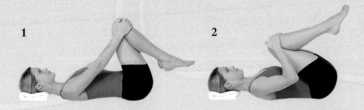

1   2

from a practitioner skilled in rehabilitation methods, such as a specialist osteopath, a physiotherapist or a chiropractor.

There are also various specific measures that can alleviate all kinds of back pain. For example, deactivation of trigger points may help considerably – consult an expert in this area, such as a neuromuscular therapist or a licensed massage therapist. Acupuncture and TENS can ease chronic back pain – although only temporarily, unless you deal with the underlying causes.

If you are suffering backache for which there is no obvious cause, use your pain diary to record the answers to questions such as: what makes the pain feel better? and what makes it feel worse? – your notes will help an expert to pinpoint the problem.

If your pain features tight muscles either side of your spine, you could try this simple exercise. Place two tennis balls in a sock and tie it off to stop them escaping. Lie on the tennis balls, so that one is on each side of your spine. By slowly moving around on the balls, you can get pressure right into the tight, sore spots that need to relax. Use this technique as often as you feel it helpful, always following up with a gentle stretch for the painful area.

Hydrotherapy can ease back pain in several ways: ice and cold ("warming") compresses relax tense muscles; alternate hot and cold applications improve circulation; and periodic ice applications reduce inflammation. Avoid hot packs, unless you follow up with massage or a cold application, as heat alone, even though it may feel good at the time, will usually lead to blood congestion.

If your pain is being worsened by inflammation, you could explore anti-inflammatory dietary strategies. If stress and anxiety are affecting you, relaxation methods, such as autogenic training, biofeedback and visualization may be helpful, too.

chest pain

Associated as it often is with heart conditions, chest pain can be worrying. However, pain in the chest is more likely to relate to the muscles between the ribs (the intercostal muscles) than to the heart. If we do not breathe properly (see pp.58–9), these muscles can develop trigger points and become highly stressed. As soon as we correct our breathing, the intercostal pain should ease. Angina pain (which usually manifests in the left arm) tends to remain unaltered, even when we breathe properly. So, if you are concerned about the cause of your chest pain, inhale deeply – if the pain changes, your heart is probably not to blame. If you are in any doubt, consult a doctor.

If you have a painful cough, try putting two drops of hyssop (or Olbas) oil into a bowl of hot water. With a towel covering your head and the bowl, place your face over the rising steam, and breathe slowly for 10 minutes.

Chest pain that worsens when you are resting may be caused by a digestive problem or inflammation, and you should seek medical advice. If you have chest pain without obvious cause and you are an asthmatic, or have had a recent bout of coughing, then you can reduce your pain through a combination of massage and other bodywork; self-applied positional release methods; and stretching. Chest pain may also derive from spinal problems – these should be checked for by an appropriate practitioner.

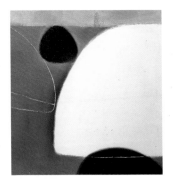

Methods that often ease pain in tense chest muscles include TENS, acupuncture, a cold ("warming") compress and any relaxation methods.

bladder, prostate and abdominal pain

If you feel a burning pain on urination you may have a **bladder infection**. Ultimately, you should seek advice from your doctor, who may prescribe antibiotics, but in the meantime, increase your fluid intake, especially water, to not less than two litres a day and take capsules of cranberry extract or drink cranberry juice (unsugared). Cranberry contains natural chemicals that help in the elimination of bacteria from the bladder. Various herbal teas, including buchu and parsley, may also be helpful.

An **enlarged prostate** may lead to difficulty in urinating, as well as aching or burning pain on urination. Seek medical advice if you are suffering from these symptoms. Taking zinc supplements, extracts of saw palmetto berries, *Pygeum africanum* or nettle root over several months may bring long-term benefit. You can derive more immediate, though temporary, relief from a prostatic massage (performed by a trained healthcare provider).

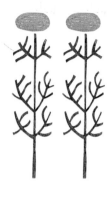

Abdominal pain can arise from so many different conditions that only general comments are possible here. These first-aid approaches should not replace responsible medical advice.

Much abdominal pain can be traced back to psychological roots. Emotional stress tends to lead to rapid, upper-chest breathing. This, in turn, means that you swallow more air, resulting in bloating and sometimes the aggravation of existing abdominal pain caused by such problems as hiatus hernia. Relaxation methods, such as progressive muscular relaxation, meditation and visualization, and slow, deep (diaphragmatic) breathing can help enormously.

Many types of abdominal pain respond well to herbal remedies. For example, the antispasmodic properties of peppermint may relieve stomach cramps. This can be taken in the form of tea, drops or capsules. Try taking ginger, chamomile, aloe vera or slippery elm (as teas, extracts or powders) to treat digestive upsets. Mastic powder (derived from a resin that is produced by the shrub *Pistacia lentiscus*) is more efficient at deactivating the bacteria that cause gastric ulcers than most antibiotics. You can ease pain relating to a spastic colon by taking aloe vera juice, slippery-elm powder (mixed into a paste with water), or charcoal capsules.

Hydrotherapy techniques provide excellent remedy for bladder, kidney and prostate problems. Try spending 20 to 40 minutes in a "neutral bath" (see pp. 74–5), or consult an expert practitioner.

A cold ("warming") compress around the abdomen and lower chest can help to soothe stomach ache and abdominal pains in general. Or you could ask your partner or a friend to massage your back or abdomen using lavender or diluted chamomile essential oil. However, ensure that you do not massage directly any inflamed tissues or organs.

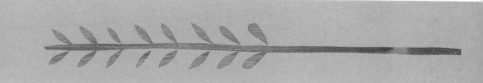

gynecological and childbirth pain

For safety, most **gynecological pain** requires medical investigation and attention. However, what follows is a brief look at some interim, self-help measures.

To ease pelvic pain and cramps, try physical and mental relaxation methods (for example, autogenic training and visualization), as well as massage, or sustained thumb or tennis-ball pressure to the lower back (see p.146). Hydrotherapy methods, such as sitz baths (see p.106) and cold ("warming") compresses on the waist (see p.107) can also help, while herbal aids include black haw and cramp bark taken as tinctures (seek advice from a qualified medical herbalist), and ginger-root tea.

Chronic pelvic pain – in men as well as in women – has been shown in many cases to be caused by trigger points in the lower abdominal and upper thigh muscles. Deactivating these points, using methods such as MET (see pp.88–91), can often eradicate the symptoms. In the USA, a group of more than 100 women suffering from chronic pelvic pain underwent trigger-point treatment. This removed all pelvic pain from 90% of the women, with most remaining pain free a year later.

If you are suffering from vaginal irritation, or pain resulting from yeast infection (thrush), try using vaginal suppositories infused with tea-tree oil or calendula; or you could mix acidophilus (a "friendly" micro-organism, available as a powder from health stores) into live yogurt and apply this mixture on a tampon. You may find that dietary and supplement strategies help – consult a qualified nutritionist or naturopath for advice.

Many non-pharmaceutical measures have been shown to help reduce **childbirth pain**. These include: giving birth in a special water tub; acupuncture; breathing techniques (especially anti-arousal breathing, see p.63); and relaxation and visualization methods. During the last three months of pregnancy, visiting a specialist osteopath once a month will help prepare your pelvis and back for childbirth, as well as easing the discomfort of late-stage pregnancy. A source of both relaxation and pain relief during advanced pregnancy is the neutral bath (see pp.74–5). To feel benefit you should spend no less than 20 minutes in the water.

Taking raspberry-leaf tea, an ancient folk remedy, for some days before and during delivery eases labour pain without interfering with the strength of your contractions.

Your birth partner can help to ease pain during your labour if they apply direct thumb pressure to tender areas of your sacrum (the bone at the base of the spine), as well as to the area on your back just below your lowest rib, close to the spine. Alternatively, you can apply acupressure yourself – try pressing firmly the tender area about one hand's width above your inner ankle bone for up to a minute at a time every half hour. The self-applied acupressure exercise described on p.138 may also help.

Bear in mind that, if you intend to use "alternative" methods (such as acupuncture or acupressure) during birth in a medical setting, you will need to discuss your plans in advance with the medical team who will be delivering your baby.

bodywide pain

Bodywide conditions demand bodywide attention – constitutional, whole-person strategies. Methods that have a calming effect on the body as a whole, such as acupuncture, relaxation massage, biofeedback, autogenic training and breathing retraining, can alleviate any of the conditions discussed here.

The causes of the chronic muscular-pain condition **fibromyalgia** are complex, often originating in a genetic predisposition, aggravated by one or more factors such as trauma, or a biochemical disturbance (for example, thyroid hormone imbalance), or a severe emotional upset. Treatment has to be very gentle indeed, to avoid placing new demands on already overloaded body systems. Strategies need to address the causes of fibromyalgia, as well as relieve the constant pain and fatigue that typify the condition. Apart from the general therapies mentioned above, you could try: thyroid hormone rebalancing (if appropriate); non-invasive manipulation methods, such as Positional Release Technique; gentle and closely monitored aerobic exercise; and sleep-enhancement methods.

The burning, tingling or aching sensations associated with **nerve pain** may derive from inflammation (neuritis), irritation or entrapment (neuralgia), or a disease of the central nervous system, such as multiple sclerosis. Other causes include infection, as in shingles, and diseases such as diabetes, cancer and arthritis.

You can ease nerve pain by taking supplements of vitamin B complex, or herbs such as passiflora, valerian or Jamaican dog-wood (but only in consultation with a medical herbalist).

A strategy known as counter-irritation may also help treat nerve pain. Try rubbing an extract of cayenne pepper onto a chronically painful area – although the skin will redden, pain usually recedes noticeably. In the case of the painful scars left over after shingles, rub in an extract of red chilli peppers. Be patient, as it may take a day or two for you to feel the benefits.

Osteoarthritis is caused by wear and tear of joints. In the early stages of the condition, you can do much to maintain good function through appropriate bodywork – stretching and move-ment – taking care not to irritate the joints. If you are over-weight, you should lose weight, as this may be placing extra stress on your joints. You can also derive benefit from hydrotherapy (for example, compresses and Epsom-salts baths) and nutritional measures, including: reducing animal-fat intake; taking supple-ments of EPA, glucosamine sulphate and chondroitin sulphate; and ingesting herbs such as devil's claw (in the form of dried, powdered root or as a tincture) and feverfew (eat one leaf a day).

The joint inflammation that characterizes **rheumatoid arthritis** can be eased by following a diet low in protein and sugar, but high in EPA (see pp.114–15). Other helpful treatments include TENS (at a high setting) and gentle exercise that main-tains muscle tone without irritating inflamed joints.

Wearing a copper bracelet can ease the pain of rheumatoid arthritis. The copper, which is absorbed through your skin, helps protect the joint membranes and joint-lubrication fluids that are damaged by the disease.

CONCLUSION: A WORK IN PROGRESS

Planning a campaign to reduce pain demands that you understand what lies at the root of the problem. By becoming familiar with the nature, causes and usual progression of your condition, you can make informed choices in terms of exercises, manual treatments, changes to your everyday activities, medication, dietary strategies, stress management and so on.

It does not matter how slowly you go so long as you do not stop.

Confucius (551–479BCE)

Having established a general plan in conjunction with someone objective and knowledgeable, such as a doctor, you need to move on to the finer points of your plan. The first thing you should do is devise your pain diary, which will be the linchpin of any project in pain management (see box, opposite). Draw up a list of action points – appointments to make with therapists or teachers, and equipment or materials to buy (for example, a TENS unit, essential oils, herbs and nutritional supplements).

So far, so good. However, you may find sticking to your plan tougher than you imagined at the initial organization stage. After a few weeks, you may start to question what you are doing. To maintain a positive outlook, give yourself a regular pep-talk – remind yourself of your objectives, set yourself challenges, congratulate yourself on every one of your achievements – no matter how small. The road to control over your pain may seem intolerably long at times, but look how far you have come already.

LOOKING BACK AND LOOKING AHEAD

Your initial pain-relief plan is by no means carved in stone. It is vital that you regularly re-evaluate all the methods that you use, dropping some, modifying others and introducing new strategies, to keep pace with your changing circumstances. Review your diary at a set time each week – look out for patterns, such as particular activities that seem to raise or lower your pain scores. Change your routine accordingly. Even methods that are working well need revisiting, and possibly revitalizing, to ensure that you do not "outgrow" them. For example:

- *Vary your relaxation exercises so that they do not become repetitive – introduce new ones or modify existing ones.*
- *Introduce fresh affirmations to reflect your evolving recovery and attitude – this will ensure that the statements continue to carry meaning for you, rather than becoming automatic.*
- *Once tight muscles have eased, you will need to modify your stretching exercises, so that they maintain, rather than increase, muscle length.*
- *As your fitness improves, you should increase the intensity of your aerobic exercises – taking care not to exceed your pulse-rate limit.*
- *If you have excluded particular foods from your diet, you should reintroduce them after six months, to check whether you have overcome your previous sensitivity to them.*

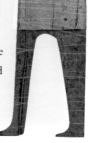

Do not underestimate the importance of your pain diary. It will become indispensable in guiding you toward your goals. As you look back, you will see what worked and what didn't – essential information in helping you decide which turning to take next in your journey toward improved health and reduced pain.

FURTHER READING

Amarnick, C.,
Dr Amarnick's Pain Relief Program,
Garrett Publishing, Deerfield
Beach, Florida, 1995

American Cancer Society,
Guide to Pain Control, American
Cancer Society, Atlanta, 2001

Benjamin, B.,
Listen to Your Pain, Viking
Penguin, New York, 1984

Chaitow, L.,
Fibromyalgia & Muscle Pain,
Thorsons, London, 2001

Davies, C. and K. N. Hardin,
The Trigger Point Therapy Workbook,
New Harbinger, Oakland,
California, 2001

Fennell, P.,
The Chronic Illness Workbook,
New Harbinger, Oakland,
California, 2001

Knaster, M.,
Discovering the Body's Wisdom,
Bantam, New York, 1996

Melzack, R. and P. D. Wall,
The Challenge of Pain,
Penguin, London, 1996
(revised edition)

Murray, M. and J. Pizzorno,
Encyclopedia of Natural Medicine,
Prima, Rocklin, California,
1997 (revised edition)

Pizzorno, J.,
Total Wellness, Prima,
Rocklin, California, 1997

Schneider, M.,
The Handbook of Self-Healing,
Arkana/Penguin, New York, 1994

Selye, H.,
The Stress of Life, McGraw-Hill,
New York, 1978

Siegel. B.,
Love, Medicine and Miracles,
Arrow, London, 1990;
HarperPerennial, New York, 1990

Woodham, A. with D. Peters,
Encyclopedia of Healing Therapies,
Dorling Kindersley, London, 1997

INDEX

ACKNOWLEDGMENTS

My thanks go to the pioneers of pain research, Ronald Melzack and Patrick Wall, and also to the army of researchers, developers and workers involved in pain management, most particularly the primary investigators of trigger points as sources of pain, Janet Travell and David Simons.

DBP would like to thank Mark Gray for his advice at the photographic shoot for this book.